# FutureDog
## Breeding for Genetic Soundness

**Patricia Wilkie, Ph.D.**

D1227702

**Minnesota Agricultural Experiment Station**
University of Minnesota — Saint Paul, Minnesota

in cooperation with the
**Canine Health Foundation**

## About the author

Patricia Wilkie has been mapping inherited diseases since 1985, working on neurological and behavioral disorders in humans before tools became available for mapping diseases in dogs. She graduated with a degree in Pathobiology from the University of Minnesota, where she was part of the Behavioral Genetics program. Returning to Minnesota in 1995, to study the inheritance of quantitative traits in livestock, she began her research on dogs.

Patricia Wilkie is currently a researcher in the University of Minnesota's Department of Genetics and Cell Biology. She has been involved in breeding Shelties since 1962 and enjoys training and showing her six Shelties in herding, conformation, agility and tracking.

## Publication notes

Production of this publication was funded by the Canine Health Foundation and the Minnesota Agricultural Experiment Station. A portion of the proceeds from its sales will be returned to the Foundation to further its activities promoting the health of our canine companions. This publication was produced through the auspices of the Communication and Educational Technology Services unit of the University of Minnesota Extension Service.

This project was supported by the American Kennel Club Canine Health Foundation. The contents of this publication are solely the responsibility of the author and do not necessarily represent the views of the Foundation.

Reference to commercial products or trade names is made with the understanding that no discrimination is intended and no endorsement implied by the Minnesota Agricultural Experiment Station or the University of Minnesota. Trademarks and trade names mentioned are the property of their respective owners.

The University of Minnesota, including the Minnesota Agricultural Experiment Station, is committed to the policy that all persons shall have equal access to its programs, facilities, and employment without regard to race, color, creed, religion, national origin, sex, age, marital status, disability, public assistance status, veteran status, or sexual orientation.

To purchase copies of this publication contact the AKC Canine Health Foundation (251 West Garfield Road, Suite 160, Aurora OH 44202 [order@www.akcchf.org or call 330-995-0807]). This will register you for receipt of periodic updates on the availability of genetic tests. Copies of this publication, without the registration for updates, can also be purchased through the University of Minnesota (Distribution Center, 1420 Eckles Avenue, University of Minnesota, Saint Paul, Minnesota 55108 [order@dc.extension.umn.edu or call 612-625-8173]). In accordance with the Americans with Disabilities Act, the text of this publication is available in alternative formats upon request to the Distribution Center.

## FutureDog: Breeding for Genetic Soundness

# Foreword

Every breeder is a keeper of the "genetic flame" for his or her breed. Every breeding decision an individual breeder makes has the potential to affect the future of the breed. For conscientious breeders, each attempt to produce quality purebred dogs includes a strong commitment to reduce inherited disease. Linebreeding, the tool largely responsible for creating the variety of dog breeds we are familiar with today, inadvertently also aggregates deleterious genes, producing disorders that may not be apparent in every generation.

These disorders often go undetected until the condition becomes frequent enough to be recognized as inherited.Generations may be unaffected when carriers are rare. As unaffected carriers become common, more affected individuals will appear. Removing affected individuals from the breeding population is not an effective solution since many unidentified carriers remain. The disease-producing genes will continue to spread unless unaffected carriers can be identified and selective breeding practiced.

***Molecular genetics creates options.*** Until recently available molecular diagnostic methods began to be used, there was little chance of eliminating all normal appearing carriers from a breeding program. This is because they could not be identified until affected offspring were produced.

***Genetic markers are helpful.*** Identifying markers close to a disease gene is very important in the process of developing an accurate diagnostic test. The closer a marker is to a disease gene, the more accurate a predictor the test will be. Although a diagnostic test can be done with only one linked marker, a test using two linked markers that closely flank the disease gene is far more accurate.

***Locating disease genes is even more accurate.*** Eventually, after markers very close to a disease gene are found, it becomes possible to actually isolate and clone the disease gene. Once this is done, a disease gene can be compared to a normal gene and a very accurate diagnostic test developed. This test is based on the actual genetic error that is inherited. The information can be used to determine if a particular dog has or does not have the error in its genetic material. If a dog does have the genetic error, it may be at risk for developing the inherited disease sometime in its lifetime.

Identification of the specific genetic error makes a highly accurate diagnostic test possible, and enables further studies to determine how the mutant gene produces the observable disease symptoms. For some human diseases, work has already progressed to this point, and many ingenious methods are being attempted to repair the genetic errors. Unlike humans, however, we will not need to repair the genetic errors in dogs because use of diagnostic tests prior to breeding will nearly always allow us to avoid producing affected dogs.

***The research process advances our understanding.*** Every research advance provides new information and improves our ability to deal with inherited disease effectively. We begin with a diagnostic test that uses only one marker. Then we move to the increasingly improved diagnostic tests as flanking markers are placed closer and closer to the disease gene. Each discovery brings us closer to the defective gene and identification of the exact genetic error. Eventually, after studying the defective gene, we can begin to understand how the disease pathology is produced, and how early intervention might modify or stop the disease process.

*Dedication*

Dedicated to:
Jilly, for the possibilities,
Ceilidh and Shad, for fulfillment,
Myst and Meidne, for perspective,
Echo and Thunder, for understanding,
Ghilly and Luna, and "the road not taken . . ."
Memories of our time together travel with me always.

***Acknowledgments.*** I would like to thank many individuals who have provided help, encouragement and advice to me during the preparation of this book. More than anyone else, Robert Kelly, AKC director and Canine Health Foundation director, has made this publication a reality by believing in it from the beginning, offering support, advice and, most importantly, working to make the information accessible to breeders, in whose hands rests the genetic future of our delightful purebred companions.

I also thank those who offered suggestions and comments on the early versions of the manuscript, especially Shauna Brummet, Ph.D., Kendall Corbin, Ph.D, Gordon Theilen, D.V.M., Asa Mays, D.V.M., Mary Galloway, D.V.M., and Pamela Peat.

Deborah Lynch, executive vice president of the AKC Canine Health Foundation, deserves special thanks for clarifications and improvements to a later draft of the text.

I am grateful to graphic artists Jim Kiehne and Dennis Bastian for rendering the illustrations into final form. Thanks also to David Hansen of the University of Minnesota Extension Service and Minnesota Agricultural Experiment Station, whose quick eye and reflexes captured most of the photographs, and to the many owners who encouraged their dogs to pose for us. Thanks to Naomi Kraus for selecting several additional photographs of performance events and to the *AKC Gazette* for providing them. Susan LaRue, D.V.M., Colorado State University, generously allowed us to include her photographs of the pseudocolorization technique in the text and as part of the cover design. Marek Switonski, Ph.D., graciously offered use of his dog karyotypes prior to publication. I am also appreciative of the effort several owners went to in providing photographs from their personal albums. Last, but not least, thanks to Minnesota Agricultural Experiment Station senior editor Larry Etkin for reviewing numerous versions of the manuscript and, finally, creatively pulling all the pieces together into the finished publication you have before you.

This publication was funded by a grant from the AKC Canine Health Foundation, and by the Minnesota Agricultural Experiment Station. It was produced by the Experiment Station with assistance from the Communication and Educational Technology Services unit of the University of Minnesota Extension Service. A portion of the proceeds from its sales will be returned to the Canine Health Foundation to further its activities promoting the health of our canine companions.

*P.W.*

# Contents

# How dog breeds began: selecting for desirable characteristics

The dog was probably the first species domesticated by man, about 100,000 years ago in southwest Asia. Ancestors of the modern wolf began to associate with primitive man, feeding on remains of hunted game and on other human leavings. Over the thousands of years that followed, groups of humans, and their increasingly domesticated wolf/dog companions, likely moved eastward and northward across Asia, eventually making their way over the Bering land bridge into North America. Along the way, their partially domesticated canine companions began accompanying other groups of humans encountered in the journey.

Descendants of the early wolf/dogs are still found today. The Australian dingo, pariah dogs of southeast Asia and the 'singing dog' of New Guinea — its name derived from its unusual vocalizations — represent the most direct living descendents of the early canines. However, even these pure ancestral types are becoming increasingly rare in the wild as they interbreed with modern domestic dogs.

## Early dogs

From the artwork of primitive man and the fossil remains found by anthropologists, a description of the ancestral type has been pieced together. This picture is of a fox-like, medium-sized dog with upright, pricked ears, a hooked tail and a short coat of reddish-tan color.

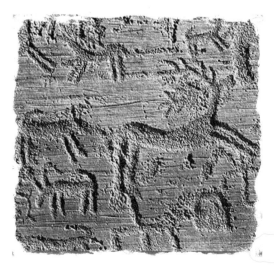

*Rock and cave paintings thousands of years old show how long canines have been helping their human companions at herding and hunting game.*

The general description of the ancestral dog could fit several modern dog breeds. Which breed it fits best can be debated because we lack distinguishing details. The details that distinguish our modern breeds have been added to the picture by selective breeding. This process has produced all of the specific characteristics that allow us to distinguish a Basenji from a Foxhound or either of these from a Miniature Pinscher or Boxer, or a Spaniel from a Keeshond . . .

## The beginning of selective breeding

When people decided to keep one dog rather than another or to acquire particular dogs with desirable characteristics, hoping to see these characteristics in the offspring, they began the process of **selective breeding**. This process is behind the tremendous variation reflected in our modern dog breeds. Whether by accident or design, as dogs with particular **morphological (physical)** characteristics became distinctive, they were also recognized for behavioral traits and for the services they began to perform for man. As particular dogs became recognized as better than average at hunting, retrieving, tracking or herding, humans selected mates for these dogs that looked similar or showed similar abilities. These breedings frequently resulted in offspring with similar or improved capabilities.

## Breeds develop

As particular morphological characteristics became more clearly associated with the ability to perform valued services, the ancestors of our present-day breeds appeared. When breeding for characteristics became more predictably associated and refined in subsequent generations, the early breed specimens began to take on what today's breeder calls **type**. In other words, *individual dogs began to resemble their more immediate ancestors and others closely related to them more than they resembled distant ancestors and dogs not closely related to them.* The inherited similarities and differences could often be observed both in physical characteristics and in particular aspects of behavior. However, the selection criteria were limited only to characteristics that could be directly observed (**phenotype**) in a dog or its offspring.

**breed;** *a group of genetically related dogs with specific characteristics which are maintained by selective breeding, are readily recognizable, and can be predictably anticipated from the matings of appropriate breeding pairs.*

**morphological;** *pertaining to the morphology or observable physical form of a particular trait or characteristic.*

**phenotype;** *the appearance or behavior of a breed or individual that can be directly observed.*

**selective breeding;** *deliberate choice of mating pairs, with retention of offspring having desirable traits for future breedings.*

**type;** *the sum total of characteristics and traits that typify a particular breed and are essential to making it distinctive from other breeds or lineages within a breed.*

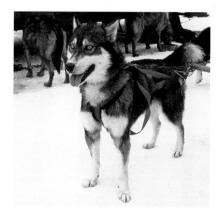

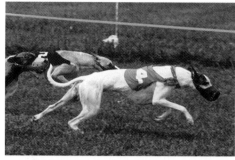

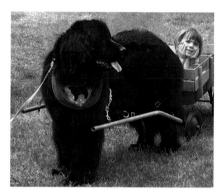

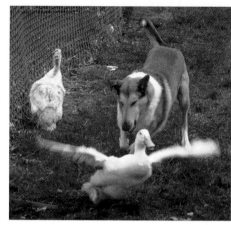

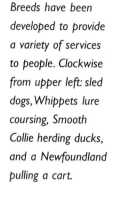

*Breeds have been developed to provide a variety of services to people. Clockwise from upper left: sled dogs, Whippets lure coursing, Smooth Collie herding ducks, and a Newfoundland pulling a cart.*

As an inherited constellation of characteristics became readily recognizable as a specific **breed** and was honed to reasonable predictability over many generations, registries such as The American Kennel Club were established to keep pedigree records. As pedigree record keeping became routine, breeders undoubtedly realized that desirable traits could often be produced more readily by breeding dogs that were related through a common ancestor.

## Linebreeding for breed type

When a breeding pair has a common ancestor that is a first degree relative, such as a parent, sibling, or its own offspring, we call the result **inbreeding**. If the common relative is more distantly related to the breeding pair, the term **linebreeding** is used.

**inbreeding;** *matings between closely related dogs, such as between first degree relatives (to parent, sibling, or its own offspring).*

**linebreeding;** *a breeding between dogs with a common ancestor, but one that is more distantly related than with inbreeding.*

# Figure 1. Illustrations of linebreeding and inbreeding.

parent/offspring mating

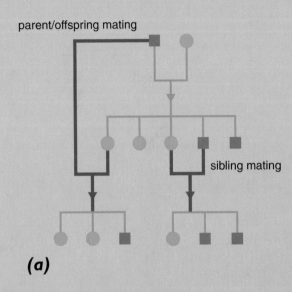

sibling mating

**(a)**

Inbreeding is the mating of first degree relatives. Sibling matings may not necessarily be littermates but could come from different litters out of one set of parents.

Blue boxes represent males.
Magenta circles represent females.

A mating pattern used extensively by some breeders ("the sire of the sire be the grandsire of the dam on the dam's side") results in pups 37.5% related to A.

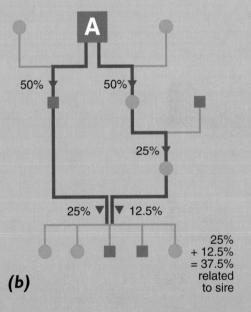

**(b)**

Linebreeding and inbreeding are similar and can be distinguished only by the degree to which the breeding pair is related through their closest common ancestor.

From a genetic point of view, the difference in degree of relatedness among ancestors of an inbred dog, as compared to a linebred dog, can be quite significant (figure 1). Linebreeding can, however, approach or exceed the degree of relatedness produced with inbreeding, particularly when a common ancestor appears many times in the recent generations of a pedigree (figure 2). You can see this by comparing the offspring illustrated in figure 1a to those in figures 1b and 2.

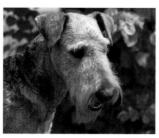
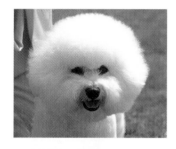
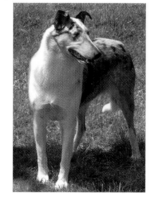
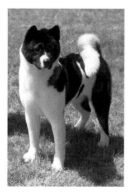
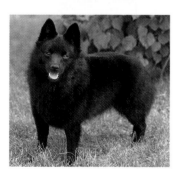
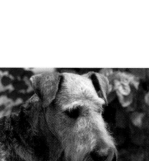

*Selective breeding has created a wide variety of dog breeds that differ markedly in appearance, temperment and ability to perform different services for their human companions. Clockwide from the upper right: Bichon Frise, Smooth Collie, Akita, Airedale Terrier, Australian Shepherd, and Schipperke.*

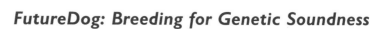

# Figure 2. Relatedness between various close matings.

In these examples, numbers indicate relatedness to sire A or dam B and could be a dog of either gender in the particular generation (dark violet pathways show lines of direct descent). All siblings in a litter have the same percent relatedness.

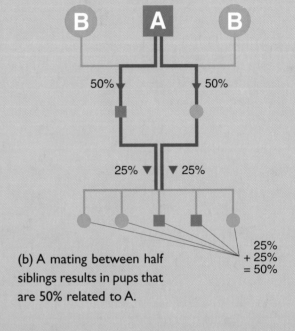

(a) A mating between full siblings yields offspring that are 50% related to A and 50% related to B.

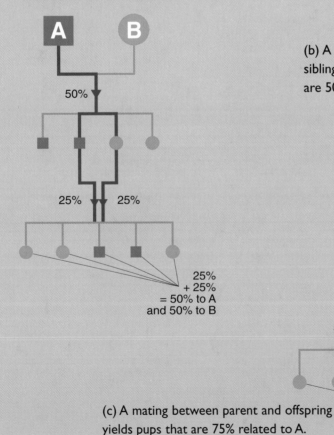

(b) A mating between half siblings results in pups that are 50% related to A.

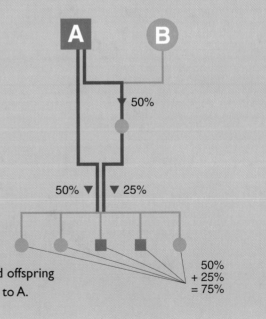

(c) A mating between parent and offspring yields pups that are 75% related to A.

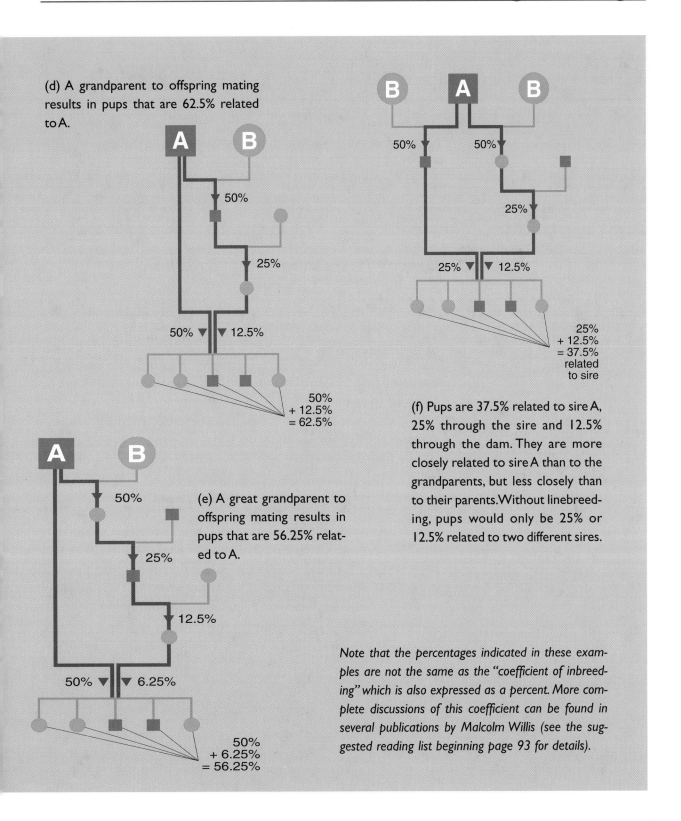

(d) A grandparent to offspring mating results in pups that are 62.5% related to A.

50%
+ 12.5%
= 62.5%

(e) A great grandparent to offspring mating results in pups that are 56.25% related to A.

50%
+ 6.25%
= 56.25%

25%
+ 12.5%
= 37.5%
related
to sire

(f) Pups are 37.5% related to sire A, 25% through the sire and 12.5% through the dam. They are more closely related to sire A than to the grandparents, but less closely than to their parents. Without linebreeding, pups would only be 25% or 12.5% related to two different sires.

*Note that the percentages indicated in these examples are not the same as the "coefficient of inbreeding" which is also expressed as a percent. More complete discussions of this coefficient can be found in several publications by Malcolm Willis (see the suggested reading list beginning page 93 for details).*

### Advantages and disadvantages of linebreeding

An important feature of these breeding techniques is that *identical copies of a gene can be inherited from the common ancestor through both parents.* If inheritance of the genes confers a desirable characteristic, this is fortunate. If the genes are deleterious (harmful), inheritance may result in disease in the resulting generation. However, it is important to note that while linebreeding was and still is necessary to set and maintain breed type; both linebreeding and inbreeding can contribute to the expression of disease-producing genes that appear naturally in the breed gene pool.

### Distant linebreeding and outcrossing

In general, it is probably more efficient to use distant linebreedings or outcrossings until the characteristics of a line are known. Closer linebreeding or inbreeding are best reserved for situations where the risk of producing affected pups appears minimal. This approach is conservative, but probably not overly so when we consider the possibility that every genetic defect will not be expressed in every environment. Some inherited diseases will be apparent only under very specific environmental conditions. Even though a dog may have the genes necessary to produce disease, if an environmental "trigger" is lacking, no disease may be observed.

### Effects of inbreeding and linebreeding

Neither inbreeding nor linebreeding can actually be blamed for *causing* disease-producing genes, but both can increase the *expression* of some of these genes by bringing undesirable genes together, concentrating them enough to manifest disease. This problem is less severe in domesticated species that have long been raised primarily for the purpose of providing a plentiful food source.

## *Differences between livestock and companion animal breeding*

In agricultural livestock production, aggressive selective breeding has traditionally been practiced to both weed out inherited disease and enhance desirable traits. Animals with desirable traits are allowed to produce young, and the less well endowed are culled from the herds. Only a few select animals raised as livestock live long enough to express the disease-producing genes that they carry. By contrast, modern nutrition and health care have extended the lifespans of our dogs.

## *Genetic testing to aid breeding decisions*

Fortunately for our companion dogs (whose life spans are frequently long enough to express disease producing genes), recent advances in genetics are beginning to allow us to make major changes. New genetic tests will increasingly make it possible for breeders to produce healthier pure-bred dogs by predicting *prior to breeding* what traits are likely to result. They may also provide veterinarians with *pre-symptomatic diagnostic information for predicting inherited disease*, so that simple changes in care or feeding routines can begin early enough to lessen the severity of an inherited disease.

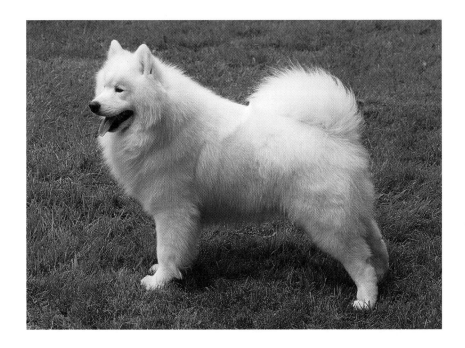

*The Samoyed, with its sturdy, muscular body and protective, joyous disposition, was bred to be a reindeer shepherd, sledge dog and household companion.*

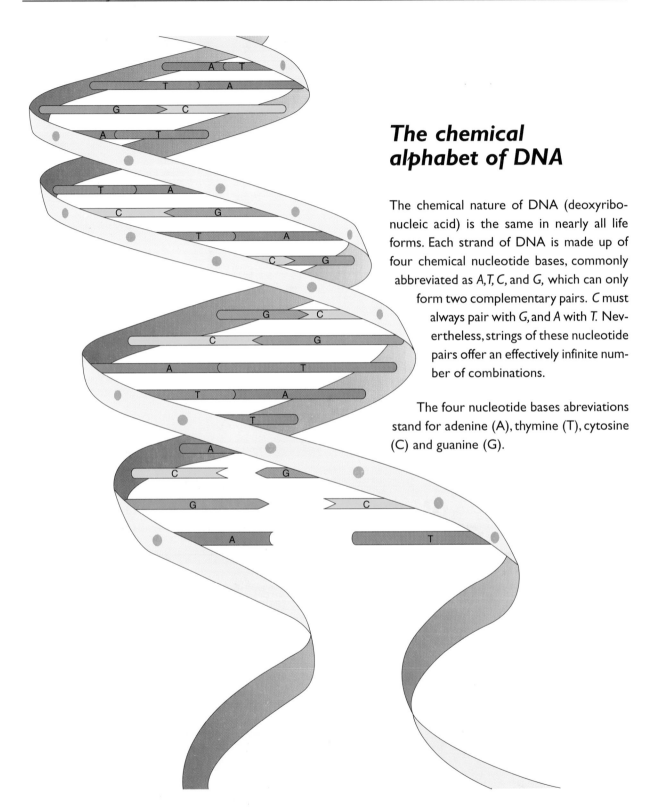

## The chemical alphabet of DNA

The chemical nature of DNA (deoxyribonucleic acid) is the same in nearly all life forms. Each strand of DNA is made up of four chemical nucleotide bases, commonly abbreviated as A, T, C, and G, which can only form two complementary pairs. C must always pair with G, and A with T. Nevertheless, strings of these nucleotide pairs offer an effectively infinite number of combinations.

The four nucleotide bases abreviations stand for adenine (A), thymine (T), cytosine (C) and guanine (G).

# Continuity of life

## The chemical alphabet — ATCG

The chemical alphabet of which life is composed is the same for virtually all life forms on earth. It's the chemical alphabet that makes up DNA.

**DNA** (its full name is **deoxyribonucleic acid**) is the genetic material found in nearly all living organisms. It specifies which characteristics an offspring will inherit from its parents. Transmitted from generation to generation, DNA is a form of chemical alphabet made of four nucleotide bases called adenine, thymine, cytosine and guanine (commonly abbreviated as A, T, C, G). These four bases are arranged in three letter "words," called codons, in different combinations like beads on a string.

The long strands of DNA spell out, or code for the order and identity of the amino acids that make up the proteins of the body. The complete sequence of the chemical letters includes the information necessary to specify the combination of characteristics we recognize as a dog, cat, human, etc.

## The genetic blueprint

All of the information necessary to produce an individual is often described as the "genetic blueprint" of the individual. Half of the "blueprint" is inherited from each parent, one half in an egg (ovum) and the other half in the sperm cell that fertilizes the egg. If both the egg and the sperm cells are produced by dogs, then a viable offspring develops into a dog because the genetic material passed on by its parents in the DNA "blueprint" encodes only the genetic information to produce a dog.

> **deoxyribonucleic acid (DNA);** the genetic material of living organisms, transmitted from generation to generation, which specifies the characteristics an offspring inherits from its parents.

*Genes are the functional units of heredity that are transmitted from generation to generation. They can be thought of as the genetic blueprint that specifies a living being.*

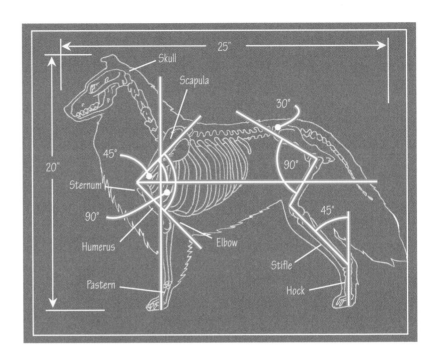

## Genes: the unit of heredity

The words of the genetic code are made up of triplets of bases joined together to form sentences that have biological meaning (i.e., they code for structural proteins in the body or catalyze biochemical reactions that are essential for life). These biochemical sentences are known as **genes.** *Genes are the functional units of heredity that are transmitted from generation to generation.* They can be thought of as a genetic blueprint that lays out the detailed characteristics of a living being.

*A dog has about 100,000 genes.* Some characteristics are specified by single genes, such as "white-factoring" present in the coat color of some breeds. For example, the color-headed white Border Collie (photo on page 23) is a result of two white-factoring genes being inherited. Were only one present, the body and head would be similar in color. Other traits require cumulative effects of multiple genes to specify a particular characteristic (for example, height at the withers).

Some genes may even influence more than one characteristic (for example, the merle coat color dilution gene also influences eye and ear development). In general, one copy of every gene is inherited from each parent, although each parent's contribution to the offspring's physical appearance or behavioral traits may not always be observable.

**genes;** *the functional units of heredity that are transmitted from generation to generation and are made up of the biochemical sequences of bases that form DNA.*

## *Genes are arranged on chromosomes*

If genes are thought of as the biochemical sentences encoding life, then chromosomes are the paragraphs organized of related gene families. Genes can be thought of as being linearly organized along the length of chromosomes.

The paragraph/chromosome analogy breaks down somewhat since chromosomes also contain genes that are not functionally related. Thus, they can not be equated with the cohesive thoughts of a well-written paragraph. It would be more like a paragraph with extra, unconnected words or sentences sprinkled throughout its length, or with occasional repeated words.

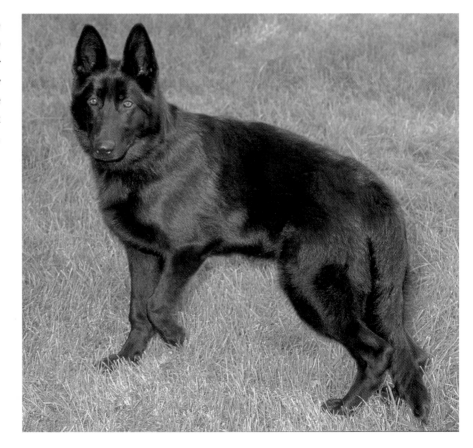

*This black German Shepherd puppy is an example of a coat color variant that appears rarely along with the more common tan and black coated littermates.*

The **genomic DNA** of dogs not only includes the biologically meaningful segments that encode genes, but also sequences of regulatory DNA and DNA with no known function. In dogs, the DNA is arrayed linearly along 78 separate chromosomes. A complete copy of the genomic DNA is present in almost every cell of an animal or plant. (The exceptions to this rule are red blood cells which lose their nucleus, and hence their DNA, as they mature).

**Dogs have 39 pairs of chromosomes.** Each chromosome has a mate that is similar in size and shape. Thus, there are actually *39 pairs* of chromosomes in dogs.

## Identifying which chomosomes are pairs

To study chromosomes in detail, dog cells can be chemically treated to stop their normal growth. The chromosomes are stained with dyes so they are spread out and are individually visible, and then a single cell is photographed (figure 3a). Each chromosome can then be cut out of the photograph and chromosome pairs matched up by their similar banding patterns (figure 3b). These matched pairs are homologous chromosomes.

## A karyotype is used to identifiy homologous chromosomes

When the pairs are identified and aligned together, the group of homologous chromosome pairs is called a **karyotype**. The karyotype in figure 3b is a picture of an incomplete set of homologous chromosomes pairs. Dog chromosomes are particularly difficult to karyotype because they are small and more similar in size than, for example, human chromosomes. Thus, only the identity of the largest twenty-one dog chromosome pairs has been agreed upon by the scientific committee charged with establishing a "common language" or standardized karyotype.

Gross chromosomal abnormalities affecting large segments of chromosomes can be detected on a karyotype and usually result in gross morphological defects that frequently result in miscarriages, stillbirths, or congenital birth defects.

**genomic DNA;** *DNA that includes more than the biologically meaningful segments that encode genes; it includes sequences of regulatory DNA as well as DNA with no known function.*

**karyotype;** *pairs of homologous chromosomes that are aligned by similar size, shape and banding pattern.*

## Figures 3a, b. Partial standardized dog karyotype.

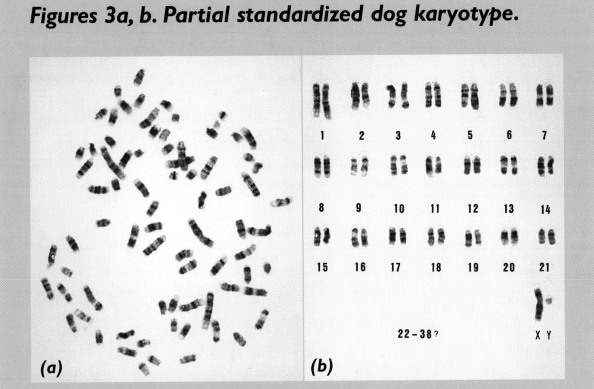

(a)

(b)

Twenty-one of the largest pairs of autosomes and the sex chromosomes (XY) can be identified using banding techniques. Those remaining of the total 39 pairs must be identified using other methods. The partial canine karyotype was generously provided by Marek Switonski, Ph.D., Agricultural University of Poznan, Poland.

## Changes in banding patterns are characteristic of some inherited diseases

Genetic errors involving missing or rearranged bands have long been recognized as hallmarks of certain cancers and congenital birth defects. Traditionally, these errors have been identified by comparing chromosome pairs that should have similar banding patterns, but in some segments do not.

### Coloring the bands makes it easier to match up homologous pairs

Special reagents or computer enhancement techniques make it possible to color the bands of dog chromosomes. These processes make it easier to match up the chromosome pairs by their banding patterns, making nearly all of the dog chromosomes distinguishable from each other.

Pseudocolorization (shown on the cover and in figures 3c and 3d) is one of the methods useful for artificially enhancing the natural banding patterns of dog chromosomes to aid finding the matching pairs and detecting errors in banding patterns that result in disease.

## Figure 3c. Pseudocolorization enhances the natural banding patterns of chromosomes.

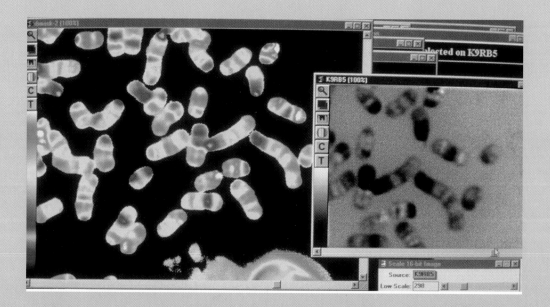

Pseudocolorization of chromosomes helps identify the homologous pairs of the smallest dog chromosomes, and detect errors in banding patterns that may result in disease.

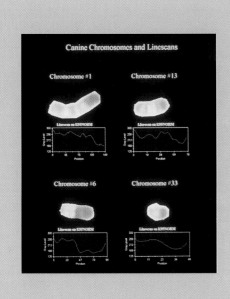

## Figure 3d. Lineal displays compare color bands with precision.

A lineal display precisely compares colors of different chromosomal bands, and makes pinpointing any changes in the large segments of a homologous pair of chromosomes vastly more simple.

However, the changes that result in normal variation in a breed or in most inherited diseases are not detectable in a karyotype. These variations must be examined at the level of the DNA. Another method, chromosome "painting," can detect errors at the level of DNA.

## Chromosome pairs are called homologs

One chromosome of each **homologous** pair is donated by each parent to an offspring. A homologous pair of chromosomes encodes the same genes in the same order, but the specific details of the gene on each homolog may not be identical.

## Polymorphism means many forms

The variation between *a particular gene and its mate* on a pair of homologous chromosomes is called a **polymorphism** (meaning many forms). The basic concept of polymorphism is important for understanding how the location of a particular gene on a chromosome is deduced and how the relative location is used to estimate the risk that any particular puppy might have for inheriting a defective gene. These methods will be described in detail after the groundwork for understanding has been laid.

**homologous;** *a pair of chromosomes that are similar in size and shape, and encode the same genes in the same order but may vary slightly in sequence of DNA.*

**polymorphism;** *the variation between a particular gene and its mate on a pair of homologous chromosomes.*

*Parental cell (showing only 2 of the 39 pairs of homologous chromosomes).*

*Replication of each chromosome to form chromatids.*

*Homologous chromosomes synapse and recombination occurs.*

**chromatid;** *two identical copies of a chromosome replicated during meiosis, each becoming a new chromosome as new cells form.*

**meiosis;** *the production of egg and sperm cells through doubling, recombination and then reduction of genetic material.*

**recombination;** *physical breakage and reunion of DNA strands that results in genetic variation.*

**synapse;** *joining of homologous chromosomes just prior to recombination in the regions where they are similar.*

Recombination results in regions of grandmaternal (shown in magenta) and grandpaternal genes (green) being arrayed together on the same chromosome. The cells produced carry either one of the possible recombinant (green plus magenta) or nonrecombinant (either totally green or magenta) chromosomes shown in the diagram and mature into egg and sperm cells.

Note the doubling of genetic material during replication, then the normal reduction of the number of chromosomes back to 39 in the egg and sperm cells. These cells will unite to form a puppy that inherits grandmaternal and grandpaternal genes present on either recombinant or nonrecombinant chromosomes.

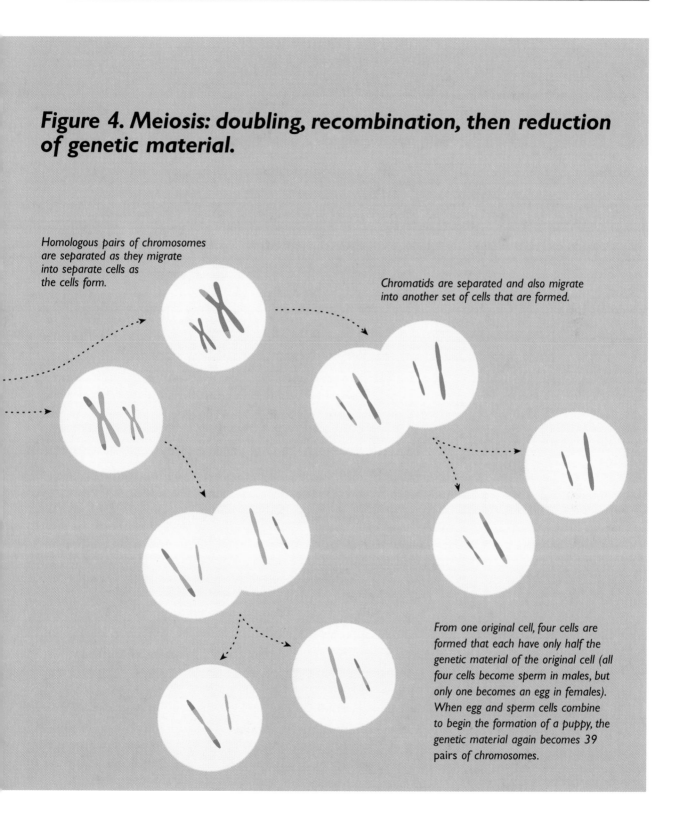

# Figure 4. Meiosis: doubling, recombination, then reduction of genetic material.

Homologous pairs of chromosomes are separated as they migrate into separate cells as the cells form.

Chromatids are separated and also migrate into another set of cells that are formed.

From one original cell, four cells are formed that each have only half the genetic material of the original cell (all four cells become sperm in males, but only one becomes an egg in females). When egg and sperm cells combine to begin the formation of a puppy, the genetic material again becomes 39 pairs of chromosomes.

## Mendelian inheritance: one gene from each parent

Of the four possible copies of a particular gene that may be inherited from a set of parents (two from each parent), only two (one from each parent) will actually be inherited by any particular offspring (see Figure 4). This pattern is know as **Mendelian inheritance**, after the Austrian monk Gregor Mendel, whose studies of the garden pea in the mid-1800s led him to postulate the basic laws of genetic inheritance.

Mendel understood that the genetic material must be transmitted as a unit with some traits inherited together and others inherited independently. However, he did not know that genes were made up of DNA and arranged linearly on chromosomes.

## Inheritance by chance: independent assortment

Which chromosome of each parental pair is received by a particular offspring is purely a matter of chance. This is called **independent assortment**. The 39 chromosomes from a sperm and the 39 chromosomes from an egg (ovum) that unite to form a puppy could differ completely between two litter mates. This is an exceedingly rare but possible occurrence. More often, litter mates will receive some copies of the same chromosomes from each parent, and on average, will share 50% of their genes.

## The sire determines the sex of each puppy

All normal dogs will have the same number, size, shape and general staining pattern of their chromosome pairs. The only exception will be found in the chromosomes that carry the genes determining the individual's sex.

*Mendelian inheritance; the inheritance of one copy of a gene from each parent by its offspring.*

In dogs, as in people, the female sex chromosome is designated X and the males sex chromosome Y. The Y chromosome carries the information regulating development of the male sex organs. Without this information the puppy develops into a female. Males have an X and Y chromosome paired together. Thus, a litter's sire determines each puppy's sex, contributing either the X or the Y chromosome to the sperm that unites with the ovum contributed by the dam (which bears one copy of either of her X chromosomes). Puppies that inherit the XY combination are males, and puppies that inherit XX are females.

# *Diversity of life*

Two normal biological mechanisms cause genetic variation. **Independent assortment** results in variation because the 39 pairs of separate packages of genes we call homologous chromosomes separate independently of one another. Just as the results of successively flipping a coin (heads or tails) are independent events, the passage into an egg or sperm of one homolog or the other of each pair of chromosomes is independent.

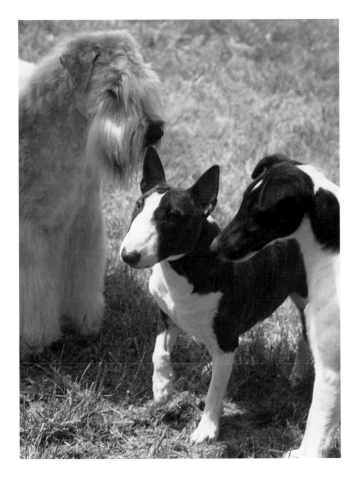

Terriers have long served humans as hunting companions and by guarding livestock and gardens from invasion by other small mammals. Different terriers have been bred for specific abilities. The Soft Coated Wheaten Terrier (left) is prized for hardy stamina, courage and tenacity. The Bull Terrier (middle), developed as a gentleman's fighting dog, is taught to defend master and self, yet not provoke a fight. The Smooth Fox Terrier (right), a quick, alert hunting breed, is skilled at driving fox from refuge.

**independent assortment;** *the random distribution of chromosomes, during meiosis, to what eventually become egg and sperm cells.*

The independent assortment of homologous pairs of chromosomes can be observed. This is because there is detectable variation or **polymorphism** among the DNA molecules that make up the chromosome pairs. If the pairs were identical, independent assortment could not be detected. Therefore, it would not make any difference to genetic inheritance because the outcome would be the same regardless of which homolog was passed on to form an egg or sperm cell.

## Eggs and sperm gametes are formed after meiosis

Formation of the **gametes**, the male's sperm and female's eggs, occurs during meiosis. Each chromosome **replicates** itself to form two **chromatids**, the identical copies that become chromosomes (figure 4). Then, homologous chromosomes line up next to one another, nucleotide for nucleotide, gene for gene, during **synapsis**.

## Recombination also produces genetic variation

The chromatids from different homologous chromosomes may exchange genetic material, including entire genes, between homologs that are in alignment. This is another mechanism producing genetic variation. This important process, the *physical breakage and reunion of DNA strands containing the genes,* is called **recombination**. It is an actual physical breakage and reunion, or swapping of genetic material between chromatids.

## A puppy inherits genes from its grandparents

The genes present on independently assorting chromosomes are inherited together in the absence of recombination during meiosis (the nonrecombinant chromosomes are entirely only green or magenta in figure 4). Thus, traits coded by these linear arrays of genes will be inherited together in a particular puppy. Which combination of grandparental genes a particular puppy inherits, from either the maternal or paternal granddam or grandsire, will be determined by whether it received a recombinant or nonrecombinant chromosome.

**polymorphism;** *the variation between a particular gene and its mate on a pair of homologous chromosomes.*

**gametes;** *the male's sperm cells and the female's eggs (ova).*

**replicate;** *when a chromosome is duplicated during meiosis.*

**chromatid;** *two identical copies of a chromosome replicated during meiosis, each becoming a new chromosome as new cells form.*

**recombination;** *physical breakage and reunion of DNA strands that results in genetic variation.*

**synapsis;** *joining of homologous chromosomes just prior to recombination in the regions where they are similar.*

When recombination occurs between genes on a chromosome (the recombinant chromosomes are shown as combined green and magenta in the figure), the linear group is broken up and the puppy receiving a recombinant gamete will have a combination of grandmaternal and grandpaternal traits for the genes on this chromosome.

*Recombination is only detectable when there are differences (polymorphisms) that are in some way observable between two genes on homologous chromosomes.*

*Many breeds are capable of perfoming, and enjoying similar tasks requiring physical skill or agility. This is illustrated in an Agility Trial competition. Clockwise from upper left: Bearded Collie, Labrador Retriever, Golden Retriever, Belgian Tervuren, German Shorthaired Pointer and color-headed white Border Collie.*

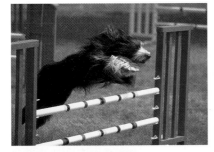
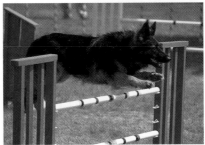
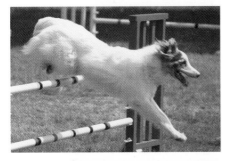
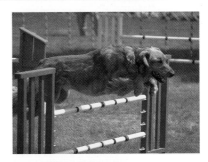
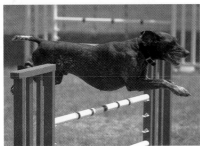
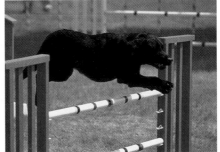

## Meiosis is the square dance of chromosomes

After synapsis, the homologous chromosomes are drawn to opposite ends of the cell by contraction of molecular threads, and a cell membrane grows between them to form two separate cells containing complementary segments of parental DNA (and, thus, homologous sets of parental genes). This first phase of meiosis reduces the total number of chromosomes in each forming gamete by one-half. In the dog, the number of chromosomes (78 or 39 pairs) present in most cells in the body, is reduced to 39 in each normal gamete.

*These Shiba Inu littermates received different coat color determining genes. The Shiba Inu breed has a more than 3,000 year history in Japan. Bred for flushing and hunting small game, today it serves as a fiercely loyal and obedient guard dog.*

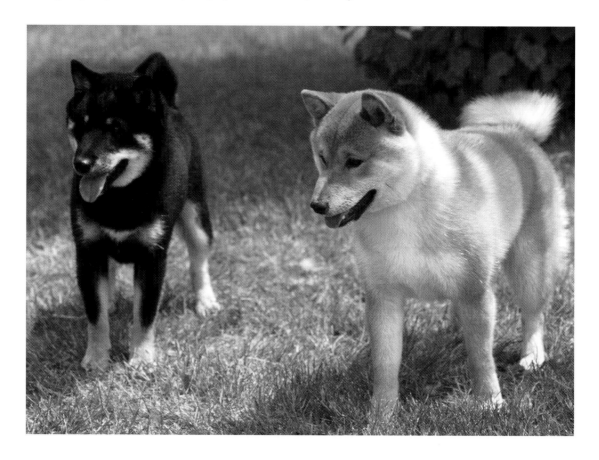

During the second phase of meiosis, another division of chromatids occurs, but with no further replication, so no recombination can occur. Then, chromatids, rather than homologous chromosome pairs, separate and move to opposite ends of the cell before another membrane grows between them to produce cells that mature into the gametes (sperm or ova) with 39 chromosomes per cell.

Figure 4 is a stylized illustration of the process of meiosis. Though only two chromosomes are shown in the diagrams for simplicity, the process described in figure 4 occurs simultaneously for all 39 pairs of dog chromosomes.

For each round of meiosis starting from a single cell, males produce four sperm and females produce one egg and three cells that do not mature into eggs. When an egg and sperm are united during fertilization, ultimately forming a puppy, the puppy will have 39 *pairs* of chromosomes (totaling 78) with one copy of each gene from each parent, just the same number as each of its parents received from the pup's grandsire and granddam.

The reduction in the number of chromosomes in a gamete is biologically sensible since it leaves each gamete with 39 chromosomes containing only one copy of the genetic material. If the reduction division did not occur, the number of copies of each chromosome would be doubled with each generation, which would rapidly become a biological burden.

## A locus is the address of a gene

Genes are linearly arranged on chromosomes. The specific place where a particular gene resides is known as the **locus**. Like the address of a house places it relative to the streets in the neighborhood and other homes on the block, the locus describes the location of the gene relative to other genes. The order of the genes is depicted on a map of the chromosome. The relative distance between genes can also be estimated from genetic data by a method known as linkage analysis. A brief description of linkage analysis begins on page 59.

*locus;* the specific location of a gene on a chromosome.

A dog receives one of each chromosome pair from each parent. Thus, it has two copies of each gene, one inherited from each parent. These genes reside *at the same locus* on a homologous chromosome pair. These two copies of the gene are called **alleles.** A dog with two identical alleles at a locus is called a **homozygote.** A dog with two alleles that are slightly different in their nucleotide sequences is called a **heterozygote,** or is said to be **heterozygous** at that locus**.**

Individuals will be heterozygous at some loci and homozygous at others. Two individuals (even litter mates) will rarely be the same over many loci unless they are identical twins.

*The Whippet was originally developed as a rabbit courser and is capable of running at speeds of up to 35 miles per hour.*

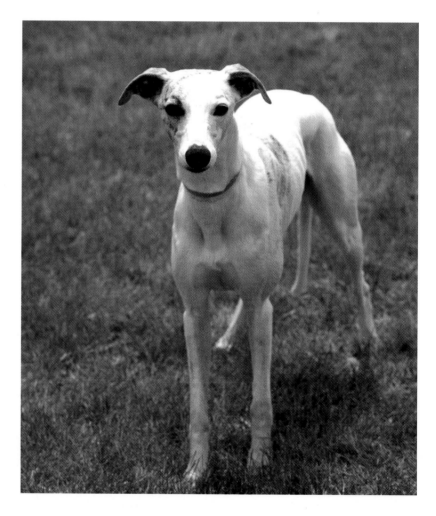

Part of the normal variation seen in a dog breed is due to the variation among alleles at a locus. For example, most breeds have several possible basic coat colors: black, red or sable, etc. These may be alternative alleles at the basic coat-color locus. In a similar manner, if any puppy inherits one or two merle alleles rather than the alternative non-merle alleles at a second coat color locus, the gene acts to produce a *diluted* coat color of either gray or red depending on the genes present at the basic coat-color locus. In this case, the gene products produced by one locus (merle) modify those produced by another locus (basic coat color), as illustrated in figure 5.

An individual dog can have only two possible gene variants (alleles) at a single locus (one inherited from each parent). However, there may be many different alleles within a larger group. A*n entire breed population may have many possible alleles at a particular locus*. When more than one possible allele exists at a locus within a breed population, the gene is **polymorphic** or has several forms. Conversely, when there is no variation at a particular locus, it is called **monomorphic** because it has only one possible form (that is, all dogs of a breed are the same).

Breeders familiar with the genetics of coat color inheritance in their breed will recognize that there is something missing from the example above. What's missing is the concept of dominant and recessive behavior or patterns of inheritance of the alleles at a particular locus.

## Dominant or recessive alleles

When two identical alleles are necessary at a particular locus to produce a particular characteristic or trait, the trait is said to be **recessive**. If only one copy of a particular gene results in the observable trait, the allele acts in a **dominant** manner.

## Environment influences gene expression

The observable result of the action of a particular gene may be influenced by the environment the dog resides in as well as by other genes it has inherited. For example, diet and exercise seem to influence the effect of the genes that contribute to canine hip dysplasia.

*alleles;* alternative forms of a gene, one inherited from each parent.

*dominant;* when the presence of only one copy of a particular gene results in an observable trait.

*heterozygote;* where two alleles that are slightly different in their nucleotide sequences are present on the respective chromosomes of a homologous pair.

*homozygote;* where two identical alleles are present on the respective chromosomes of a homologous pair.

*monomorphic;* no observable variation at a particular locus, i.e. it has only one possible form.

*polymorphic;* when more than one possible allele exists at a locus within a breed population.

*recessive;* when two identical alleles at a particular locus are required to produce a particular characteristic or trait or disease.

## Figure 5. Inheritance of variation at two coat color loci.

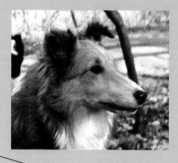

*Gametes possible from a bifactored sable merle male with a genotype BcMm*

*Gametes possible from a bifactored tricolor female with a genotype bcmm*

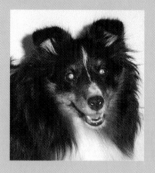

|  |  | BM | cm | Bm | cM |
|---|---|---|---|---|---|
| bm |  | BbMm | bcmm | Bbmm | bcMm |
| cm |  | BcMm | ccmm | Bcmm | ccMm |

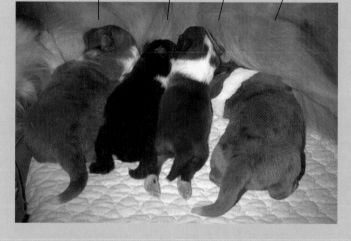

**incompletely penetrant;** *when a particular gene is inherited but the phenotype expected is not expressed (observed).*

In some inherited diseases, the sex of the affected dog seems to modify the severity of the disease symptoms. When a particular gene is inherited but the phenotype expected is not expressed (observed), we say that the gene is **incompletely penetrant**. A dog that

## An example of a trait influenced by more than one gene.

Here the base coat color locus (sable or black, **B** or **b**) and the color modifying locus (merle or nonmerle, **M** or **m**) interact to produce the coat color.

In the example, **B** represents the sable coat allele, **b** the black or "trifactor" coat of black with tan points, **c** the "bifactor" or black coat without tan points, **M** the merle or coat dilution factor and **m** the undiluted coat allele. A dominant allele (**B** at the base coat color locus; **M** at the merle color modifying locus) inherited from one parent and a recessive allele (either **b** or **c** at the base coat-color locus or **m** at the merle locus) inherited from the other parent will result in the **phenotype** of the dominant allele being observed in the puppy.

The recessive allele inherited from the other parent will not be evident. (In the example, **B** is dominant over **b**, **b** is dominant over **c** and **M** is dominant over **m**). Although the general rule applies across all breeds, which colors are dominant will vary by breed. In some breeds black is dominant over other coat colors.

A "Punit square method" (shown in the example to the left) can be used to figure out the proba-ble frequency of each type that will result in the progeny of a particular mating. This method can be used for all loci that are due to inheritance at a single gene locus, whether the gene encodes a normal or disease trait. (The more complex case where multiple genes interact to produce a trait is discussed in greater detail on page 38.)

It is customary to give the same symbol to the alleles at a single locus. Usually, the dominant allele is indicated in upper case and the recessive in lower case letters, although many different notations and symbols have been used. With complex inheritance patterns, it is often necessary to modify the notation.

*Punit Square Abreviations:*

| | | |
|---|---|---|
| BbMm | = | trifactored sable merle |
| BcMm | = | bifactored sable merle |
| bcmm | = | bifactored tricolor |
| ccmm | = | biblack |
| Bbmm | = | trifactored sable |
| Bcmm | = | bifactored sable |
| bcMm | = | bifactored blue merle |
| ccMm | = | biblue merle |

inherits a disease gene but does not show the disease phenotype, (i.e., the gene is incompletely penetrant) can often pass on a completely penetrant disease gene to its offspring.

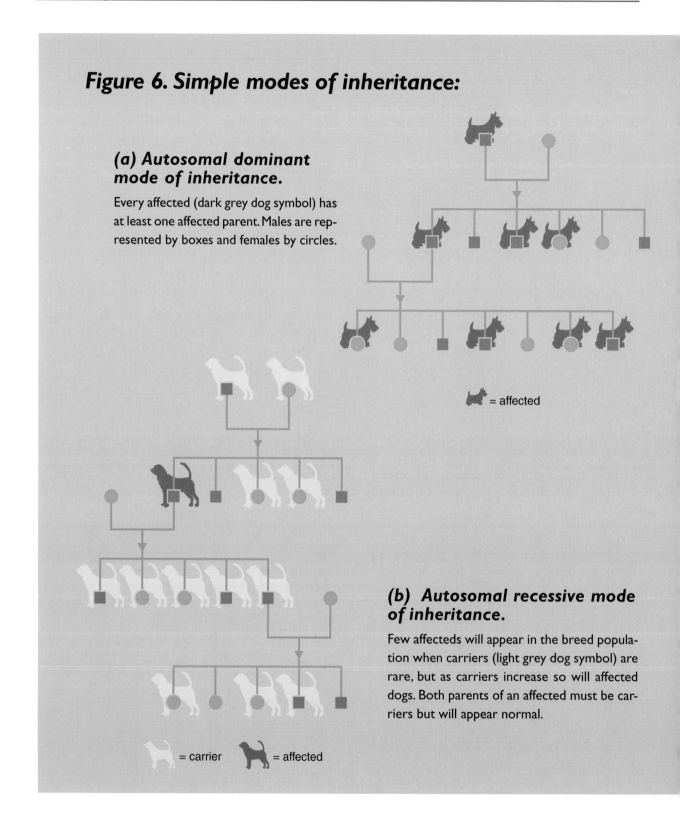

# Figure 6. Simple modes of inheritance:

## (a) Autosomal dominant mode of inheritance.

Every affected (dark grey dog symbol) has at least one affected parent. Males are represented by boxes and females by circles.

= affected

## (b) Autosomal recessive mode of inheritance.

Few affecteds will appear in the breed population when carriers (light grey dog symbol) are rare, but as carriers increase so will affected dogs. Both parents of an affected must be carriers but will appear normal.

= carrier   = affected

## (c) Sex-linked mode of inheritance.

Carriers appear normal and can not be detected until they produce an affected offspring, unless a diagnostic test has been developed to detect them [the bold **X** denotes the sex chromosome that encodes a disease producing gene].

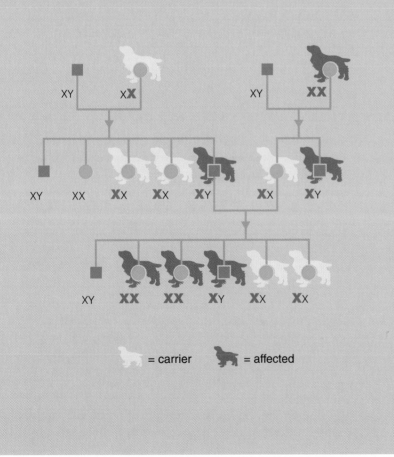

# To test your understanding . . .

Try to draw a square for each nuclear family in figure 6c and compare the genotypes you obtain with the diagram. The correct answers are at the bottom of this page.

Can you explain why the lower family has two affected and two carrier *female* pups, when only 25% of the offspring should be affected and carrier females, respectively? (See "lower" Punit square below.)

The mating was drawn this way to illustrate how the predicted ratios of offspring of each type are only estimates for a large sample of the breed and may vary either way, producing an excess or lack of any type where only a small sample, such as the litter here, is considered. When data for many litters are gathered, the observed ratios should conform to the predicted ratios.

If breeders suddenly recognized a disease was inherited, were able to recognize affected and carrier dogs, and then chose not to breed a particular type (such as affected or carrier males or females), a comparison of the frequency of each type before and after should reveal a decline in the numbers of affected and carrier offspring corresponding to the lack of breedings involving these genotypes.

You can determine for yourself by drawing the Punit squares, the projected make-up of the breed population when only affected dogs are eliminated from breeding, compared to eliminating both carriers and affected dogs from the breeding population.

In figure 6a, for a dominant gene with a test to identify affected animals, if none are used for further breeding, a disease is eliminated in one generation.

For figure 6b, eliminating affecteds and carriers from breeding stock means the disease is also eliminated in the next generation. Carriers can be safely bred to a mate that is known to be normal because it has been tested, though in this case half of the offspring would be expected to be carriers.

Similar exercises can also be done for coat color inheritance of the Collie pups on page 58. (See Punit squares on page 58.)

You can see from these exercises that even crude diagnostic tests capable of identifying presymptomatic affected and carrier dogs can be powerful tools not only for decreasing inherited diseases but for achieving more rapid success in breeding top-quality dogs for any trait the breeder desires.

---

*Answers for 6c:* (**XY** = *diseased male;* **XX** = *diseased female;* xy = *normal male;* **X**x *or* xx = *normal female*)

| **upper left** | ♀ | x | **X** | | **upper right** | ♀ | **X** | **X** | | **lower** | ♀ | **X** | x |
|---|---|---|---|---|---|---|---|---|---|---|---|---|---|
| ♂ x | | xx | **X**x | | ♂ x | | **X**x | **X**x | | ♂ **X** | | **XX** | **X**x |
| Y | | xY | **XY** | | Y | | **XY** | **XY** | | Y | | **XY** | xY |

## Mode of inheritance: single gene traits

The first step in understanding any specific genetic trait is to identify its mode of inheritance.

## Dominant inheritance

If incomplete penetrance is not a factor in the expression of a particular gene, a dominant gene generally will be observed in every generation of a pedigree (figure 6a). Thus, every affected dog will have at least one affected parent. If there is only one affected parent, on average half of all offspring will show the trait.

## Recessive inheritance

A recessive inherited trait will appear to skip one or many generations because it will not be observable (expressed) without two like genes present at a locus. Individuals that have inherited only one recessive allele are *carriers of the trait*. The mating of two carriers of the trait may produce disease in some of the puppies who inherited a copy of the recessive allele from each parent (figure 6b).

*The Siberian Husky was bred for endurance to be a sled dog. This husky has inherited a mutation that causes two different eye colors (one brown and the other blue). This appearance is accepted in the breed standard.*

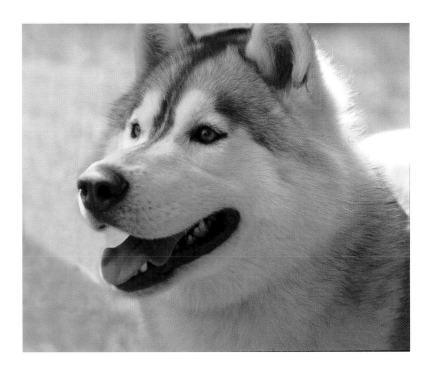

When the trait in question confers an inherited disease, and carriers are rare in the breed population, the frequency of the disease will also be rare. Recessive disorders are insidious because when the disease is rare in the breed population, the number of carriers will increase gradually in the absence of testing to detect carriers and selective breeding of only animals that are not carriers for the trait. Eventually, carriers of the trait may become quite common in the breed, particularly if the trait is located on a chromosome near enough to a desirable trait to be inherited along with it frequently.

As the number of carriers increases in the breed population, so too will the numbers affected by the disease. This mechanism is similar for the spread of recessive traits across the breed population, whether the trait is desirable or undesirable.

*Dalmatians served as coach or carriage dogs. Inherited deafness is common in the breed.*

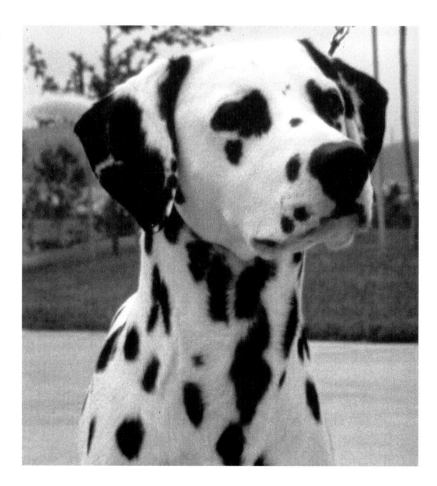

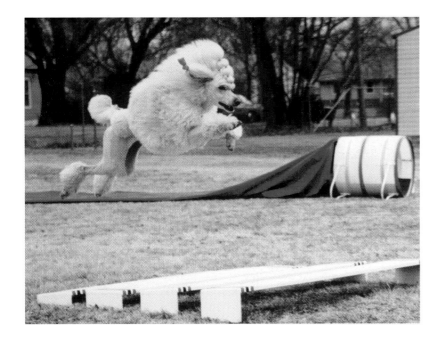

*The Standard Poodle originated as a water retriever, and its classical shorn appearance was derived from a desire to facilitate the animal's swimming. The natural intelligence of the breed makes it a strong competitor in agility events.*

## Sex-linked genes

A gene showing sex-linked inheritance confers a trait that appears only in one sex, unless affected dogs are used for breeding (figure 6c). The genes for most sex-linked traits are found on the X chromosome, since the Y chromosome seems to encode few genes.

A female pup will inherit an X chromosome from each parent. She in turn, can pass on a copy of either X chromosome to her pups of either sex. However, a male pup can inherit an X chromosome only from his dam and a Y only from his sire, and can pass on his X chromosome only to his daughters and his Y only to his sons. A trait inherited in this manner usually appears to be transmitted through only one sex (dams) and inherited by only one sex (male pups)(figure 6c family at upper left).

The exception to this rule is rare. An affected male mated to a carrier female (who will appear normal) (figure 6c family at lower middle) or an affected female mated to an affected male (not shown), can produce affected females. Unless this happens, disease will occur only in the sons of carrier dams because female litter mates will have one normal copy of the gene. Half of the daughters of these dams will also be carriers and all daughters of affected males will be carriers.

Breeding affected dogs of either sex is risky. However, breeding a male affected with a sex-linked disease to a known normal female (not shown) is far less serious than breeding an affected female to a known normal male (figure 6 at top right). Note that the same method illustrated in figure 5 can be used to calculate the genotypes and likely frequency of each genotype in this example.

## *Mode of inheritance: polygenic traits*

Traits with dominant, recessive or sex-linked modes of inheritance are generally termed simple or single gene traits because they involve a single gene locus. The inheritance of both normal variants and disease traits can be observed to show simple patterns of inheritance. A trait can also be determined by the action of genes at two or more loci. This pattern of inheritance is termed **polygenic** or complex inheritance. Polygenic inheritance can be thought of as a group of genes acting together in concert to produce a particular phenotype.

Most traits influencing conformation and behavior, for example hock length, height or "eye" shown when herding stock or the posture shown by many hunting dogs, are probably determined by the action of genes at multiple loci.

**polygenic;** *a complex inheritance pattern that can be thought of as a group of genes acting together to produce a particular phenotype.*

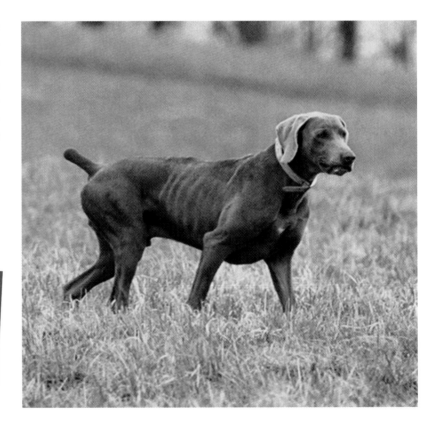

## Figure 7. Normally distributed curves for two quantitative traits.

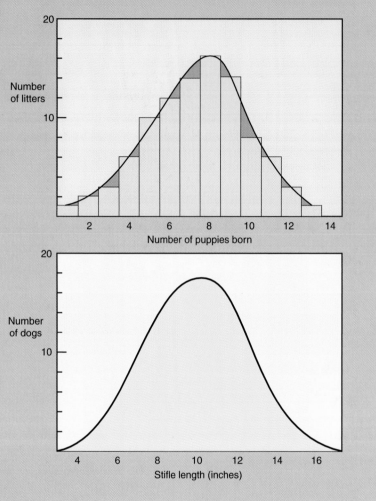

The histogram beneath the curve in the upper graph is made by simply counting the number of puppies born in each litter and plotting against the number of litters born. This plot represents a breed that has an average of 8 puppies per litter.

Likewise, a trait such as stifle length can be measured and plotted against the number of dogs which have each length stifle. The plot in the lower graph represents a breed that has an average stifle length of 10 inches.

Polygenic inheritance of a trait is usually suspected when none of the simple patterns of inheritance are observed in pedigrees followed over several generations. There are statistical methods for identifying polygenic traits. These are routinely used to locate quantitative or polygenic traits of economic importance in domestic livestock populations. These same methods will undoubtedly be used to search for genes encoding polygenic traits in dogs.

A trait is suspected of being polygenic if it shows a range of measurements in a population. When the trait values are plotted on a graph against the number of individuals with each measurement, a bell-shaped curve or normal distribution is obtained. This curve form describes situations where there are many individuals in the breed population with middle or average trait values and fewer individuals that measure at either of the extremes (figure 7).

## Inheritance patterns of polygenic traits

Polygenic traits can be inherited in a *dominant* manner similar to simple dominant traits except that multiple loci each contribute to the trait phenotype. For example, suppose loci P, Q and R contribute equally to the phenotype of length of the upper front leg bone (humerus) which markedly influences the front angulation of a dog. Dogs inheriting any combination of the genotype, including a large P, Q and R (e.g., PPQQRR, PpQQRR, PpQqRr, etc.) will have the same length bone (assuming that the environment does not influence bone growth). However, dogs inheriting combinations of lower case or recessive alleles at a locus (eg., ppQQRR, ppqqrr or PpqqRr, etc.) will have a shorter bone length. The number of loci with only recessive alleles will determine how short the bone will be.

Polygenic traits can also be inherited in an *additive* manner when the alleles at each locus contribute, regardless of which combinations are present. In this case, the length of the humerus bone discussed above would be determined simply by the *total number of upper case alleles* in a genotype. For example, the order of bone length from largest to smallest for the combinations shown would be PPQQRR, PPQqRR, PPQQRr, PpQqRr, ppQqRr, ppQqrr where 6, 5, 4, 3, 2 and 1 upper case alleles, respectively, contribute to the phenotype of bone length.

A third possibility for a trait showing polygenic inheritance requires the presence of a particular allele at one locus in combination with specific alleles at other loci. This mode of polygenic inheritance is called an **epistatic effect** because an allele at one locus influences the expression of other loci. This situation is extremely complex.

**epistatic effect;** an allele at one locus influencing the expression of another locus.

**mutation;** a biological mistake that introduces variation into a genome which can be harmful, favorable or have no apparent effect.

*Individuals of some breeds, such as this Briard, have double rear dew claws which are thought to be inherited in a dominant manner. In fact, the Briard breed standard requires that they be present, placed low on the leg, giving a wide base to the foot and, ideally, forming additional functioning toes. They are an example of an advantageous mutation. Fewer than two dew claws on each rear leg is a disqualification in the breed ring.*

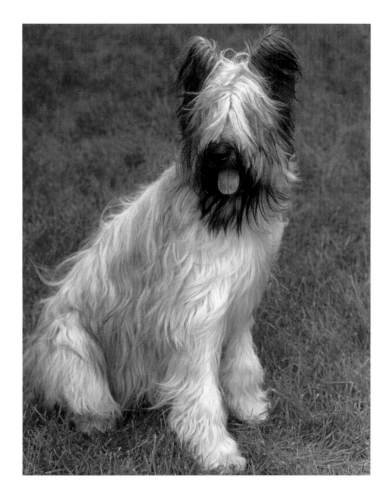

The prediction of offspring phenotypes from genotypes is impossible unless the major loci involved in producing a particular trait phenotype are known. It is also clear that a trait determined by a few genes, say three or four, is more amenable to prediction of offspring phenotype than a trait determined by hundreds of gene loci that individually contribute small effects to the phenotype.

## Mutations: how inherited diseases arise

Genes usually are transmitted faithfully from parents to offspring. A biological mistake made in this process produces another type of genetic variation: a **mutation**. Only mutations that have occurred in the formation of cells destined to become gametes can be inherited by future generations.

Mutations can be harmful (causing disease), neutral (having no effect) or favorable (resulting in an enhanced characteristic). When a new dominant mutation occurs, particularly one that is not observable until after maturity, when it may already have been passed on to offspring, it can spread rapidly through a breed population. This is particularly true when the mutation is inherited by a popular sire, who has the opportunity to pass the gene on to many offspring. If the mutation improves a particular characteristic, so much the better; but if it results in disease, breeders are likely to be plagued by it before they even realize it has a genetic cause.

### Not all new mutations produce disease

Mutations are a necessary part of any change whether the change is disease producing or desirable. Most mutations probably do not occur in sequences coding for genes, so will not affect a dog's observable characteristics.

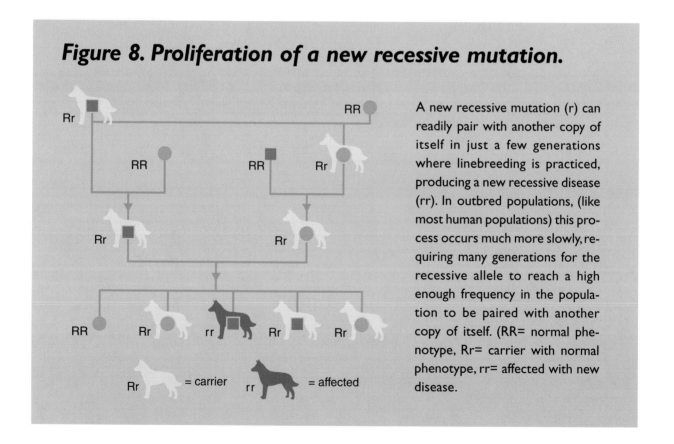

## Figure 8. Proliferation of a new recessive mutation.

A new recessive mutation (r) can readily pair with another copy of itself in just a few generations where linebreeding is practiced, producing a new recessive disease (rr). In outbred populations, (like most human populations) this process occurs much more slowly, requiring many generations for the recessive allele to reach a high enough frequency in the population to be paired with another copy of itself. (RR= normal phenotype, Rr= carrier with normal phenotype, rr= affected with new disease.

# What a breeder can do.

When linebreeding is used to set and maintain breed type, it is possible for a new recessive mutation to be paired with an inherited copy of itself in offspring. This will spread a new disease in just a few generations (figure 8). If a mutation arises in or is inherited by a popular sire or dam, the mutation can become prevalent in the breed over the course of only a few generations.

How can a conscientious breeders guard against an undesirable gene arising in or being introduced into their lines? If an affliction appears multiple times in a lineage, the assumption may be made that it could be genetic. In the past, little could be done except to avoid breeding affected dogs or dogs that produce affected pups.

Dealing with an inherited disorder in this manner is time consuming. It also allows numerous opportunities for a disease-producing gene to be passed on to offspring before a dog that carries a deleterious gene is detected.

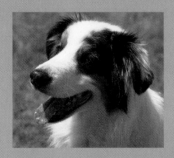

*Australian Shepherd*

Fortunately, new technology developed originally to aid in detection of human disease genes is now being adapted for use with dogs.

For a few inherited diseases, it is already possible for breeders to detect carriers and/or dogs destined to become affected (e.g., copper tox-icosis in Bedlington Terriers; von Willebrand's disease in Manchester Terriers, Doberman Pinschers, Shetland Sheepdogs, Poodles, Pembroke Welsh Corgis, and Scotties; and PRA in several breeds). Efforts to develop DNA-based tests for many more inherited canine diseases are underway.

These new methods make it possible to identify both recessive disease gene carriers and those destined to be affected with late-onset dominant diseases among litters of young pups. The DNA-based tests provide several advantages over traditional breeding practices:

1.  The tests can be applied early in life, so only the most genetically fit individuals can be retained for breeding before major investments of time and energy are expended on the pups.

2.  Recessive disease gene carriers can be identified prior to breeding, so *pups destined to be affected by recessive diseases need not even be conceived.*

3.  Known carriers with otherwise superior traits can be used judiciously for breeding, because they need never produce an affected pup, and carrier pups with less desirable traits need never be bred but can live normal lives.

By using these new tools, a breeder can rapidly eliminate late-onset dominant, recessive and sex-linked disease genes from a line.

The vast majority of all mutations occurring in coding regions are known to be deleterious. These mutations must continuously be removed from the breeding population. When the variation for a particular characteristic in a breed is lost, any change, positive or negative, is impossible.

*In some strains of the Newfoundland sub-aortic stenosis, a constriction of the aorta, is relatively common. It decreases the working ability of this powerful but gentle and loyal water rescue dog. The gene that causes cystinuria, a disorder characterized by excretion of large amounts of cystine in the urine and recurrent urinary stones, has been identified in this breed.*

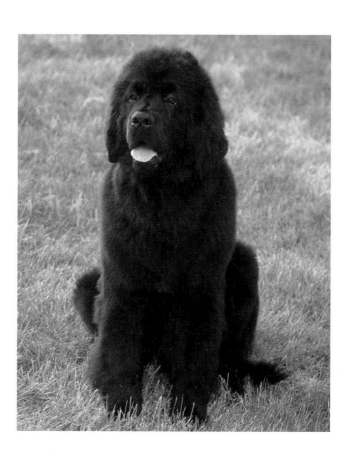

## Keys to success for improving the genetics of dog breeds.

The breeder is at the forefront of any progress that can be made in improving the genetics of dog breeds. The Parent Breed Clubs, especially, are an essential resource for organizing efforts to determine which diseases are most prevalent and most destructive in a particular breed. Our ability to detect the most destructive diseases early in a puppy's life will have the greatest impact for making informed decisions about the genetic future of the breed.

When the breed variation is limited, it becomes difficult to select effectively for desired characteristics. For example, in a breed where the majority have undesirably short tails that do not reach to the hock joint, it will be difficult to breed for improved tail length because only a subset of the few individuals with longer than average tails may be outstanding or acceptable in other characteristics.

To breed better and healthier dogs successfully, we must:

1.  Learn to manage the variation brought about by mutations that accumulate naturally within the breed.

2.  Be alert for inherited disease traits in addition to the desirable traits we seek to propagate.

3.  Honestly and openly *compare observations with other breeders to identify inherited diseases before they become prevalent in the breed.*

4.  When diseases do appear we must *work together to define their mode of inheritance.*

Only when these tasks have been accomplished, can scientists begin to look for markers that can be developed into diagnostic tests to identify carrier and presymptomatic dogs.

## Microsatellite markers are useful for mapping dog genes

One type of mutation has repeatedly occurred over the course of biological history, providing convenient and readily detectable genetic markers. This is known as a **microsatellite** polymorphism. A **marker** can identify the same specific and unique location in the genetic material of every dog. Microsatellite polymorphisms are very useful as markers because they both occur frequently and are highly variable.

Hundreds of canine microsatellite markers have already been identified. Each microsatellite marker has its own specific address in the map of every dog's genome. Using a map analogy, currently we know only the equivalent of the street address for most of the dog markers, not the city, county, state, etc. But we do know that the address can identify only one unique location and work is progressing rapidly to determine the location of dog markers, both relative to each other and by chromosome (that is, to locate them on a **genetic map** of the dog).

**genetic map;** a map showing the location of genetic markers relative to each other and genetic distances between markers.

**marker;** a reliable identifier of the same specific and unique location on genomic DNA.

**microsatellite markers;** short tandem repeats of nucleotide sequences also known as short tandem repeat polymorphisms (STRP).

Fortunately, markers need not be mapped to be useful in the early stages of work directed at ultimately producing a diagnostic test for an inherited disease, or for predicting what trait will be inherited, if these characteristics are produced by the action of a single gene (simple inheritance).

*The Belgian Malinois is closely related to three other Belgian sheepherding dogs and has been crossbred with them at several times in the breed's history.*

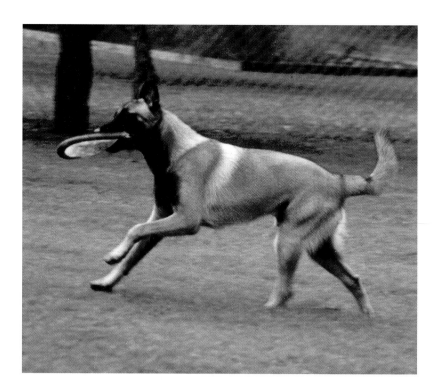

## Markers can help identify candidate genes

Markers located near genes of interest can be detected by using statistical methods to examinine pedigree data. It is likely to be rare, but not impossible, that a marker located close enough to, or within, a disease gene to become part of a diagnostic test could be found by chance or by examining candidate genes that result in somewhat similar disease phenotypes in other species (most often human chromosomes, since most genetic mapping has been done there).

It is more likely that a marker fairly distant from a disease gene would be found first. Then, detailed maps of the region would be prepared, and the position of the disease gene located between the markers on the detailed map.

## Microsatellite markers help find disease genes

*Microsatellite markers are made up of repeats* of the nucleotide bases that make up DNA and are flanked or *bracketed by unique DNA sequences*. Each particular combination of unique flanking sequences occurs at only one locus in each dog's genetic material, ensuring that the each marker has only one address.

In theory, the repeat region could be comprised of any combination of the four bases that make up DNA, but in fact, some combinations occur more frequently. Which repeats occur most frequently can vary dramatically by species. Generally, the most common repeats are made up of (CACACACA...).

Markers with larger numbers of repeats are the most likely to be polymorphic between individuals. The repeat motif involving only two base nucleotides (CACACA...or ATATAT... etc.) is called a dinucleotide repeat, but trinucleotide (CATCATCAT...) and tetranucleotide repeats (ATGGATGGATGG...) are also found often enough to be useful. Trinucleotide and tetranucleotide repeat polymorphisms are particularly prized because they are often easiest to interpret correctly.

Microsatellite repeat polymorphisms are detectable because two dogs may have different numbers of the repeat motif. A particular dog may have different numbers of repeats on each of its homologous chromosomes. This makes it possible to determine which parent contributed each copy of the repeat (unless both parents have the same genotype).

A careful examination of figure 9a will show that the pups in the litter at the bottom of the pedigree received different band lengths. (Bands toward the top of the page represent a larger number of repeats than those nearer the bottom). Bands of each size are always traceable back to the parent that donated them, with one coming from each parent. Examining the bands of the parents would confirm that they also inherited one band of each size from each of their parents.

# Figure 9a, b. A three-generation dog pedigree and evaluation of a recessive disease inheritance.

### Three-generation pedigree of dogs with corresponding genotypes for a completely informative marker

The rectangle below each individual in the pedigree shows the two alleles inherited by that individual as would be seen on an autoradiogram. Notice that the inheritance of the marker alleles can be traced through the pedigree. The standard sizes are at the left in base pairs, and the genotype of each individual is shown at the bottom of the figure in base pairs.

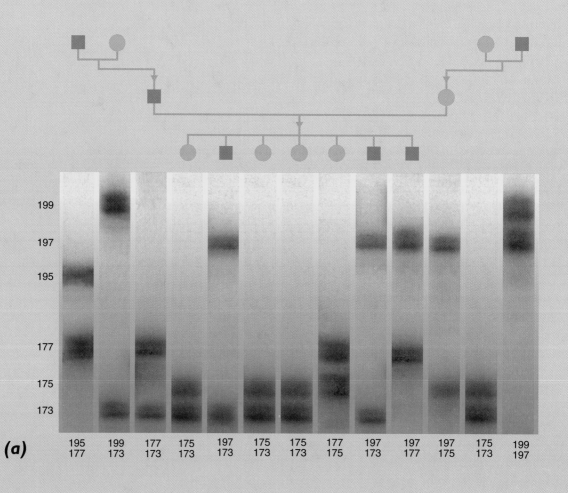

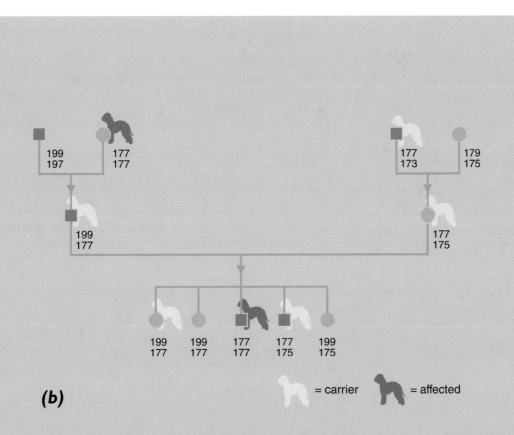

**(b)**

= carrier     = affected

### *Inheritance of a recessive disease segregating with the same marker as shown in the figure on the left (allele sizes in base pairs)*

Note that allele 177 segregates with the disease gene in this kindred. Remember that for most recessive diseases, we would not be able to identify the carriers without a diagnostic test, since they would appear normal.

After the affected male in the litter showed signs, we would know that both parents must be carriers and that one dog in each pair of grandparents must also be carriers (or affected as shown by the paternal granddam here). Without a diagnostic test, we would not know which grandparent was a carrier (unless they had produced affected offspring in other litters), so couldn't apply the information to other litters of their offspring (half siblings of the parents in this pedigree).

# To test your understanding . . .

Refer to figure 9b. Why do the female littermates (to the left) of the affected male (in the the bottom row of offspring illustrated in the diagram on page 47) inherit allele 177, but not show signs of disease? The answer is that they have only one disease allele (177). They would need to inherit two disease alleles to show signs.

Assume that all the carriers in the pedigree in figure 9b were identified as such because they produced affected offspring in other litters. The new diagnostic test for this disease using the linked microsatellite marker confirmed that these dogs were carriers, and also predicted that the female in the bottom row, second from the left (199, 177 genotype) would also be a carrier. How can this be explained?

The explanation for this circumstance is that she has produced only two litters, both by the same sire that is unrelated to her, and neither litter had affected pups. It was just not recognized that she was a carrier without the use of the diagnostic test. The sire has produced ten litters by other females and never produced an affected pup, so he is not likely to be a carrier because the disease is fairly common in this breed.

The mating was drawn this way to illustrate how the predicted ratios of offspring of each type are only estimates for a large sample of the breed and may vary either way, producing an excess or lack of any type where only a small sample, such as the litter here, is considered. When data for many litters are gathered, the observed ratios should conform to the predicted ratios.

Years later, looking back at several pedigrees, including the one illustrated in figure 9b, we notice that after the upper right dam in this pedigree produced seven litters of entirely disease-free pups, she produced an affected pup. The diagnostic test using microsatellite markers did not predict she was a carrier. What went wrong?

The linkage diagnostic test it must be remembered, can not be 100% accurate. For 100% accuracy (assuming no laboratory errors or a disease that shows incomplete penetrance—see page 28), a direct test is needed where the disease producing mutation is actually observed by sequencing the gene of each test subject.

Accuracy of a linkage test is limited by genetic distances between the diagnostic marker(s) and the disease-producing gene. The closer a marker to the disease gene, the less likely a recombination will occur between the loci to make the prediction incorrect in a few recombinant individuals. As markers used in the linkage diagnostic test are found that are closer to the disease gene, the test becomes more and more accurate, and the problem encountered in this question, failure to identify a carrier using a linkage diagnostic test, becomes less and less likely to occur.

The reason the dam in this example produced so many disease-free pups before finally producing an affected one is that carriers of the disease were rare in the breed population during most of her reproductive years. The carriers increased rapidly in the breed because a famous sire that produced over 100 champions turned out to be a carrier. Breeders were not concerned with the problem because the famous sire had never produced any affected offspring until recently.

The sire was tested as soon as the new linkage diagnostic test was available and found to be a carrier. Now breeders are testing all his descendants when doing even distant linebreedings, to avoid producing affected offspring by never breeding carriers to carriers.

The most conscientious breeders only breed known carriers to noncarriers and only then when the carrier has characteristics that are outstanding enough to warrant producing litters half of which will be carriers. By doing this, they avoid spreading the disease gene in the population, so that when they want to breed an outstanding carrier dog, there will be many noncarriers left in the breed population to choose among for an appropriate mate. If they bred carriers indiscriminantly, even to noncarriers, they would soon have few noncarrier mates available.

*The Keeshond was known primarily as a barge dog in its native Netherlands. It is believed to be derived from the same ancestors that produced the Samoyed, Chow Chow, Norwegian Elkhound, Finnish Spitz and Pomeranian.*

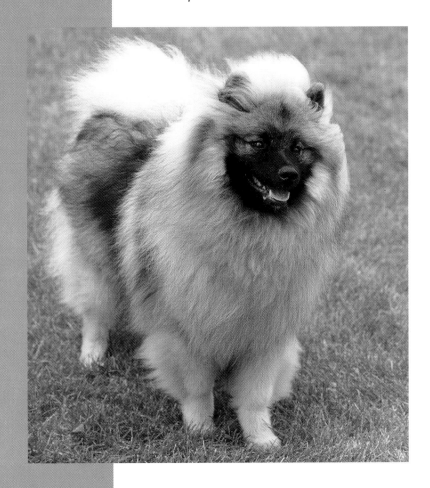

If the microsatellite marker being examined is polymorphic enough (i.e., there are enough *different* alleles in the family we are examining), we can see which parent and grandparent contributed every band to each puppy. In the situation shown in panel 9a on page 46, bands of each puppy can be unambiguously assigned to the grandparent that contributed them.

In this case, we say that the marker is completely **informative** in this family, giving us the maximum amount of inheritance information possible. Panel 9b (page 47) on the other hand, depicts a family where it is not possible to tell which puppy bands come from which parent because both parents have band 177. When there is only one puppy band we must assume that both parents contributed alleles with the same number of repeats. This marker is less informative in this family. We expect that there will be some differences in marker informativeness between families, but the most useful markers will be those that are informative in most families.

## Breed variation in marker informativeness

How informative a particular marker is will vary by breed since dog breeds are totally separate genetically due to registration requirements. *Because of this separation, purebred dogs no longer share a common gene pool, meaning that mutations that change the number of repeats in a marker will not be inherited across breeds.* The presence of similar-sized bands in two dog breeds is due either to a common progenitor (i.e., the two breeds arose from a common stock somewhere in their genetic history), or the similar band sizes arose independently in the two breeds.

Mutations that result in microsatellite polymorphisms are fairly frequent for reasons that are not completely understood. Fortunately, unless a mutation is in a functional gene, it is unlikely to cause disease. Most microsatellite markers are not believed to be within functional genes. Their utility lies in the ease of their detection in any dog, their high degree of polymorphism, and the fact that it can be readily determined if they reside near a gene of importance by using genetic mapping techniques.

**anticipation;** *earlier and earlier onset in successive generations afflicted with an inherited disease.*

**informative;** *a marker that provides the maximum amount of inheritance information possible.*

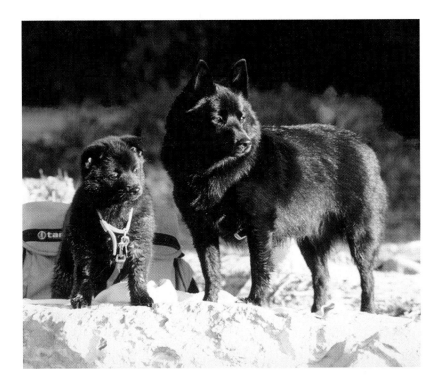

*The Schipperke's close undercoat keeps it warm in snow and dry in rain. The breed is known for its ability as a guard dog and its fondness for children.*

## Age of disease onset may be a clue

Although most microsatellite markers probably are not a part of functional genes, several have been found to be a part of a disease-causing gene in human inherited neurological diseases. All of these diseases result from major increases in the number of trinucleotide repeats present in the repeat motif, a circumstance where the length of the repeat can expand with each successive generation. An interesting clinical characteristic of these diseases is that they show earlier and earlier onset in successive generations afflicted with the disease.

Geneticists have called this successively earlier onset phenomenon **anticipation.** Anticipation was thought to have no biological cause, being simply associated with more careful monitoring of affected families once an inherited disorder was identified. Since the genes causing some of these diseases have now been isolated (cloned), it has become apparent that regions of repeat motifs are highly vulnerable to expansion and contraction mutations. In families with several affected members, the number of trinucleotide repeats in each person correlates with the severity of disease.

### Severity of disease expression

Individuals most severely afflicted with the disease usually have the largest repeat motif expansions, corresponding with the most abnormal protein product produced from their genes. Those with the least severe disease have repeat expansions that are closer to the normal number. Thus, whenever the clinical observation of variability in expression of the disease among family members is made along with successively earlier disease onset, the possibility of a trinucleotide expansion mutation is raised. It is likely that this type of mutation also is found in other mammalian species, including dogs.

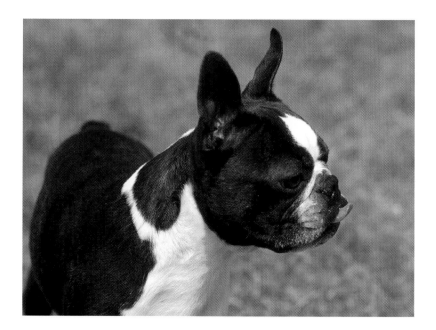

*The Boston Terrier, despite its name, is a member of the AKC non-sporting group. It was bred in the United States as a companion animal.*

# Creating genetic maps with molecular markers

Unique DNA sequences bracketing microsatellite repeats ensure that each marker has its own unique address among the thousands of bases that make up the genomic DNA. This circumstance is used to select sequences that contribute to the creation of genetic maps.

Small stretches of unique sequence DNA are selected from the bracketing regions. The complement of these stretches—remember that nucleotide base *A* always pairs with *T*, and *C* always pairs with *G*—is synthesized by chemically hooking the bases together to form **oligonucleotide primers** (the unique sequences are usually about 20 bases but are depicted as only three bases long in figure 10). The complement is required to make a primer because it is the nature of DNA that, given the right temperature and salt conditions, complementary DNA sequences will find each other with incredible accuracy and bind together to form double-stranded DNA. This property of DNA is useful because the regions between the bracketing DNA can then be **amplified** or chemically duplicated billions of times to provide larger samples for analysis (as shown in steps 3 and 4 of figure 10).

Copying the bracketed DNA is done using an enzyme commonly known as Taq polymerase. This enzyme is particularly useful because it can withstand near-boiling temperatures for relatively long periods. In its natural habitat, the bacteria from which the enzyme is obtained live in bubbling hot springs like those in Yellowstone National Park.

With the Taq polymerase enzyme and a pair of oligonucleotide primers that bracket a microsatellite repeat region, the vast complexity of the genomic dog DNA is far less daunting.

**amplified;** *copying of a section of DNA chemically billions of times.*

**oligonucleotide primers;** *small stretches of unique sequence DNA selected to flank a tandem repeat sequence that are used as primers for amplifying the segment of DNA contained between them.*

We can find a specific marker locus at will in any individual dog's DNA, make billions of copies of it and compare the number of repeat motifs between dogs to see if they are the same or different. More importantly, we can trace the inheritance of the DNA segment in multiple generations of a dog pedigree as shown in figure 9. The process that allows us to examine the genomic DNA in this minute detail is know as the **polymerase chain reaction** (abbreviated **PCR**) and is illustrated in figure 10.

Polymerase chain reaction or PCR is a series of chemical reactions used to make billions of copies of specific fragments of genomic DNA. In this process, called amplification, the fragment copied is selected by PCR primers that are specific for unique sequences on the genomic DNA. These primers bracket a series of tandemly repeated bases that are highly variable between individual dogs. The amplified region is called a marker because it "marks" a location that is found only once in the genomic DNA of each dog.

Sizes of amplified DNA fragments can be readily examined by sorting them using a process called **electrophoresis**. This process creates an image of the DNA sorted into identifying bands. Figure 10b illustrates one method where electrophoresis has been used to separate amplified DNA into peaks increasing in size from left to right.

The electrophoretic banding pattern characterizing the DNA of a dog is called a **genotype,** and the process by which a genotype is produced is often called genotyping. A set of genotypes for multiple loci is sometimes referred to as a **DNA profile** or fingerprint. A DNA profile is usually made from a set of approximately 10 highly polymorphic markers. Figure 10b shows data for only six marker loci. One can also imagine, by examining figures 9 and 11, how a DNA profile might look when using the radioactive labeling method.

If the markers used to create a DNA profile are polymorphic enough in an individual, the combination of banding patterns will be as unique to the individual as a fingerprint. DNA profiling can be used to identify an individual dog with great certainty at any time over the animal's lifetime because its DNA profile does not change. It can also verify the parentage of a dog by comparing a its profile to that of its parents, confirming parentage when half of the DNA bands of an offspring are identical to those found in each parent (figure 11).

**DNA profile;** also known as a "DNA fingerprint;" a composite of a set of approximately a dozen highly polymorphic genetic markers that characterizes the individual uniquely.

**electrophoresis;** where fragments of amplified DNA produced by PCR (polymerase chain reaction) migrate through a gel matrix, sorted by size into bands.

**genotype;** the genetic constitution of an individual that is characterized by a marker or a banding pattern at a particular locus.

**polymerase chain reaction (PCR);** the process used to amplify a segment of DNA to provide billions of copies.

## Figure 10a. The polymerase chain reaction (PCR).

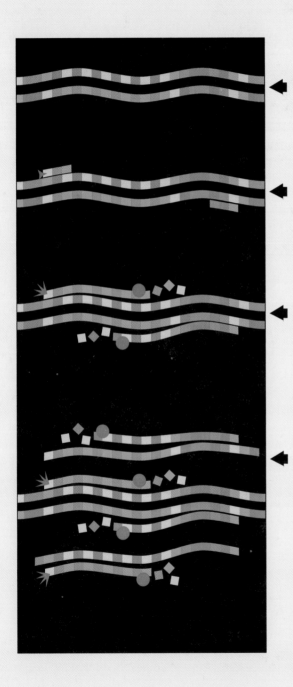

**STEP 1–** PCR is a series of chemical reactions catalyzed by Taq polymerase in which double-stranded genomic dog DNA is first denatured, or melted at high temperature into single stranded DNA.

**STEP 2–** The temperature is lowered to allow the oligonucleotide primers (shown as short segments of DNA) to find their complementary sequences on the genomic DNA (known as annealing). Every blue base pairs only with its magenta complement (representing nucleotide A paired with T), and every green pairs only with yellow (representing G paired with C).

**STEP 3–** Taq polymerase (red circle) actively synthesizes the complement of the genomic DNA between the primers (represented by the boxes joining onto upper and lower strands.

**STEP 4–** This process is allowed to occur over and over, typically thirty or forty times. The number of copies of the DNA bracketed by the primers expands exponentially to the billions.

As the DNA copies are made, they are labeled either by the incorporation of bases that are radioactive or by the use of fluorescent tags on the primers (red flare).

# Figure 10b. Electrophoresis makes DNA bands visible.

In electrophoresis, DNA fragments or PCR products are loaded onto a very thin matrix that has the consistency of gelatin and acts as a sieve. The DNA fragments wiggle through this matrix attracted by an electrical charge at the far end of the gel matrix. Larger fragments are held back by the matrix more than smaller fragments, effectively sorting them by size.

As DNA fragments are sorted across the gel matrix, if they have been fluorescently tagged in advance they can be detected as they pass by a spectrofluorometer to create the readouts shown here. The electronic image is transferred to a computer and interpreted.

Alternatively, when the fragments have been radioactivity labeled, the gel matrix containing the DNA fragments can be carefully transferred and dried onto a piece of filter paper by the application of heat and vacuum. The result can then be used to expose x-ray film, leaving banding patterns for interpretation, as in figures 9 and 11.

The DNA from many dogs can be readily compared, with similar results, by using either method.

This example shows genotypes of six markers for the sire (top), pup (middle) and dam (bottom). The size of the DNA fragments are shown at the top of the printout in base pairs. The standards (red) are in the same position in all three printouts. Each marker is tagged with a different fluorescent color (yellow, green or blue) so multiple markers can be electrophoresed at one time.

Note that the puppy will inherit one allele for each marker from each parent.

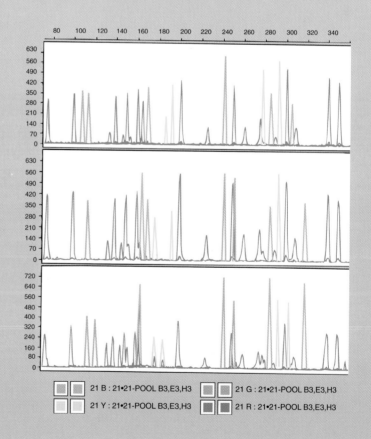

# Figure 11. Markers can be used for identifying individuals or verifying parentage.

The upper set of genotypes supports parentage with all offspring bands found in either the dam or sire. (The ▶ symbols point to the sire's contribution and ◀ point to the dam's contribution).

The lower figure shows genotypes at the same marker loci with only a partial match to the sire for pups 3 and 4. This result would be expected if the actual sire was a close relative, such as a brother or son of the sire of record. Bands with "**x**" could not be contributed by the sire of record, but could be contributed by the sire in the upper figure. You can see this by comparing the upper sire's banding pattern with pups 3 and 4.

This sire of record and the actual sire share half their bands, as would siblings, or parent and offspring. If only marker C were examined, the sire of record would not be excluded as the sire of the entire litter. Exam-

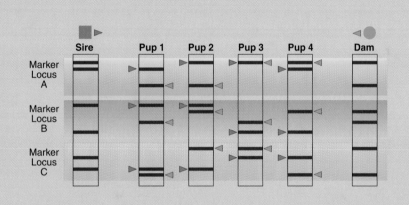

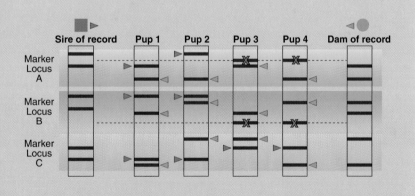

ining additional loci makes it possible to distinguish the correct sire. Even more marker loci would need to be examined to exclude or prove the sire of record was the sire of pups 1 and 2.

In general, the more informative a set of markers is, the fewer the number of markers needed to reach a prespecified threshold of confidence for accepting or rejecting parentage.

## To test your understanding . . .

Are the dams of the two litters shown in figure 11 the same or different dogs? They are different because they have different DNA profiles. Since these markers are highly polymorphic in this breed, we can see that the dams may be closely related because they have the same genotype at marker loci B and C, differing at only locus C by one allele.

This is an example of why markers that are not very polymorphic in a population will be poor at distinguishing between individuals. Many individuals in the population will have the same marker alleles (bands), especially where intensive inbreeding and linebreeding have been practiced. Markers that have low polymorphism or are monomorphic in a breed will obviously have reduced utility as tools for identifying individuals and verifying parentage. It also diminishes their usefulness as markers for detecting disease genes or desirable traits.

To overcome the problem of reduced variability in markers, more of them must be used for individual identification or parentage verification. Unfortunately, use of poorly informative markers will mean a lower chance of detecting a linkage between a marker and the gene of interest, and even if a linkage is found, the marker may not be particularly useful for diagnostic testing in many families.

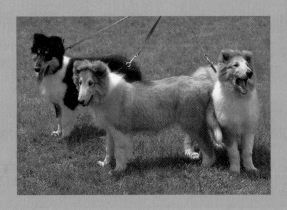

These Rough Collie pups received different coat color determining genes. Both parents must carry at least one tricolor gene and one parent must be sable coated to create this litter. The other parent could be tricolor or sable. Can you draw Punit squares for the two possible matings that could produce this litter? (See answers below.) Trifactored sables (Bb) and pure-for-sables (BB) have sable coats that may vary in sable color richness. Tricolors (bb) will all have black coats with tan points on muzzle, eyebrows and legs.

Answers:   Sable gene is dominant over trifactor gene (B = sable gene; b = trifactor gene). Pup coat colors are: BB = sable; Bb = trifactored sable; bb = tricolor.

|  |  | Tricolor Parent | |  |
|---|---|---|---|---|
|  |  | **b** | **b** |  |
| Trifactored | **B** | **Bb** | **Bb** | 50% Bb |
| Sable Parent | **b** | **bb** | **bb** | 50% bb |

| Both Parents Trifactored Sable |  | **B** | **b** |  |
|---|---|---|---|---|
|  | **B** | **BB** | **Bb** | 25% BB |
|  |  |  |  | 50% Bb |
|  | **b** | **Bb** | **bb** | 25% bb |

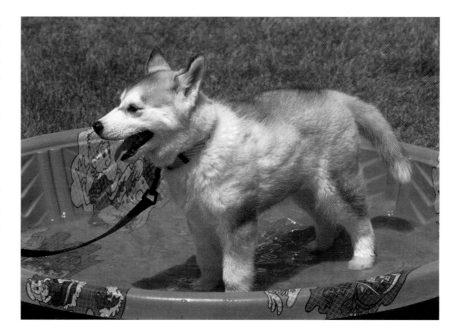

*This Siberian Husky pup reminds us that diagnostic tests using genetic markers linked to inherited disease genes will enable breeders to "clean up the gene pool" for many breeds in just a few generations if used conscientiously. With diagnostic tests it will be much easier to breed for desired traits in coming years, without having to breed around inherited diseases.*

## Mapping disease or desirable genes is the same

Recombination events make it possible to map markers to a particular location on the dog genome. Mapping is the genetic equivalent of finding the country, state, county, town, and street address of a locus (marker or gene).

The simplifying assumption underlying the creation of genetic maps is that recombination events are evenly spaced along the chromosome. Thus, when a breed population is examined, two loci that are close together have, on average, fewer recombination events between them than two loci that are farther apart (figure 12).

## Linkage is the probability of loci traveling together

By genotyping a family of dogs with several markers, and calculating the number of recombination events between pairs of loci, the distance between loci can be estimated and their "linkage," the probability of their being inherited together, can be statistically estimated. The unit of measurement applied to the analysis is the centiMorgan.

**centiMorgan (cM);** *closely related to a "recombination fraction," a measurement of the genetic distance between a pair of loci which tells us how likely it is that they will be inherited together on a single piece of nonrecombinant DNA.*

The *genetic distance between loci is a function of the probability of recombination between them. It can be thought of as a measure of the strength of the genetic linkage between loci or the probability that they will be inherited togethe*r. When genetic distance information has been obtained for a set of multiple marker pairs, this information can also be used to give us the relative order of the marker loci.

Linkage cannot usually be detected for distances approaching the recombination fraction of one-half, so we describe such loci as unlinked. For two very closely linked loci the recombination fraction approaches zero.

## "CentiMorgans" measure the distance between pairs of loci.

The unit of measurement applied to the analysis of genetic linkage is the centiMorgan. It is named after the geneticist who realized the utility of this method for statistically estimating genetic distance.

By convention, one percent recombination (also called a **recombination fraction**) be-

tween a pair of loci is called a **centiMorgan** (abbreviated **cM**). One cM is roughly equal to 1 million base pairs of DNA.

Figure 12 shows how recombination events can be detected only in heterozygous individuals, where an odd number of recombination events has occurred between marker loci.

## Genetic maps show the order and distance between loci

Linkage analysis is used to determine the distance and order of markers and genes on the chromosomes. Once the relative order and distance between loci is known, the result is called a **genetic map.** In essence, a genetic map gives a complete address of a marker or disease locus.

**genetic map;** *a map showing the location of genetic markers relative to each other and genetic distances between markers.*

New marker loci can always be added to a genetic map (if they are sufficiently polymorphic) by genotyping the families used for making the original map. This process uses the new and old marker genotypes to make estimates of the genetic distances between the new marker and the markers already on the map.

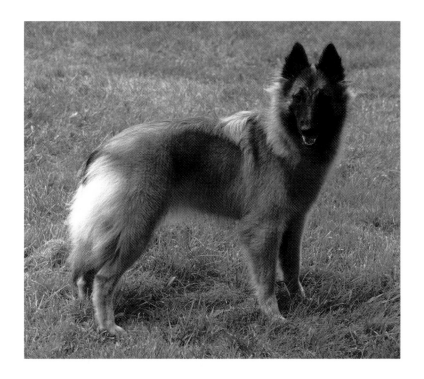

*This one-year-old Belgian Tervuren is likely to mature into an adult with a disposition well suited to be a therapy dog or companion to the disabled. They are also very versatile, participating successfully in agility, herding, tracking and obedience performance events. The breed was originally developed as a general purpose herding and guard dog. The Belgian Tervuren is closely related to the Groenendall (which has a long black coat), Malinois (with a short coat), and wirehaired Laekenois.*

## Linkage analysis measures the distance between loci

Estimating the genetic distances between loci (which can be either markers or a marker and disease gene) is known as **linkage analysis**. Although linkage analysis was invented in the early 1900s, only since the recent availability of high-speed computers has it been practical to use it for building genetic maps and for finding markers linked to inherited disease genes for the purpose of developing diagnostic tests.

The concepts behind linkage analysis are very simple. However, as one might suspect from the requirement for high-speed computers, linkage analysis can require a great deal of computation time. The basic underlying conclusion of linkage analysis is that accuracy of prediction increases as markers are found closer to the sought-after genes.

*linkage analysis; a method invented in the early 1900s for estimating the genetic distances between loci.*

# Figure 12. Breakage and reunion during meiosis

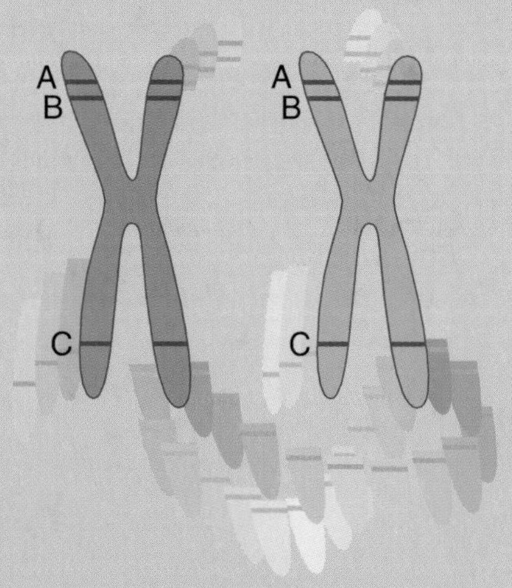

Breakage and reunion during meiosis (leading to formation of egg and sperm) results in exchange of the genetic material (DNA) between chromosomes of maternal (magenta) and paternal (blue) origin in the normal process called recombination (also shown in greater detail in figure 4). Loci that are close together (A and B) are not separated by recombination as frequently as loci that are far apart (B and C).

*process of recombination*

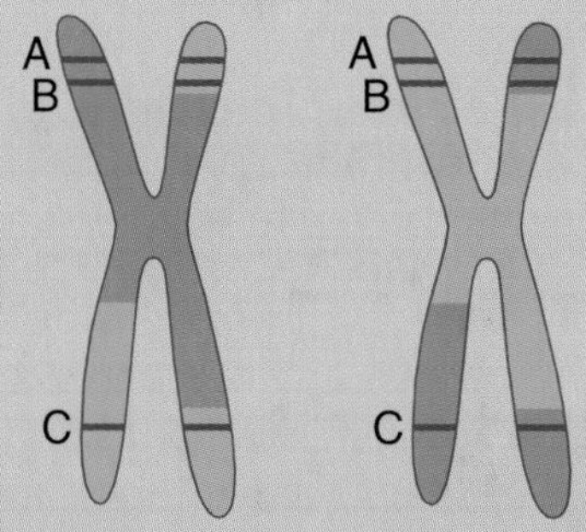

*recombinant chromosomes*

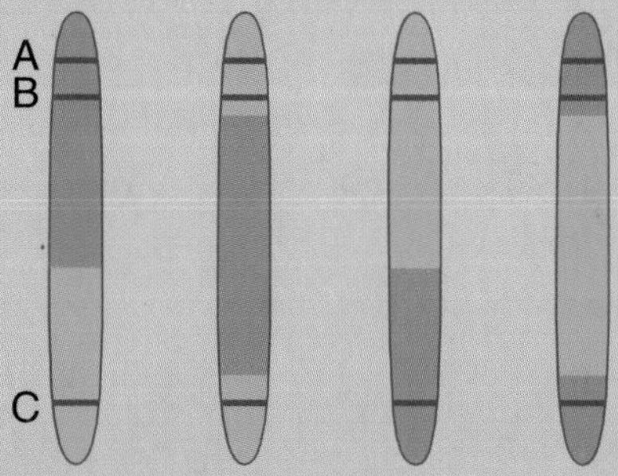

# Finding linked markers: difficult first steps to diagnostic tests.

The concept of linkage and the measurement of centiMorgans are important to the use of molecular markers as predictive diagnostic tests for the inheritance of disease-causing genes.

Though it may almost seem contradictory to say this, there is a simplifying assumption behind the complex concept of linkage analysis. This assumption is that recombination events are *evenly distributed* over the entire genome, also implying even distribution over each chromosome.

Two loci that are close together on a chromosome will necessarily have fewer recombinations between them than will two loci that are far apart. Figure 12 is a simplified example of this concept.

Suppose locus **A** and locus **B** were separated by a genetic distance of 23 cM. This would mean that recombination occurs between them approximately 23% of the time (sometimes written as a recombination fraction of 0.23). The recombination fraction is often designated with the Greek symbol *theta* ($\theta$), (as in the notation "$\theta = 0.23$").

If we assume that the genetic distance between loci **B** and **C** is 50 cM, this would correspond to an approximate recombination fraction of 0.50. Obviously, the physical distance between locus **A** and locus **B** is smaller than the distance between **B** and **C**, so we would expect a greater number of recombination events to be detected between locus **B** and locus **C** than between **A** and **B**.

If locus **B** were a disease gene and **A** and **C** were equally informative markers, **A** would be a better predictor of what allele is inherited at the disease locus from each parent than would be locus **C**. This is because **A**, being closer to **B**, would have fewer recombination events in a population sample between **A** and **B**. Therefore, in a population, **A** and **B** would travel together without being separated by recombination a higher percentage of the time than would **B** and **C**.

Thinking about it a different way, the probability that **A** and **B** would be inherited together on a contiguous piece of DNA that has not been broken up by recombination is far greater than the probability that **B** and **C** would be inherited together. Thus, marker **A** would be a more accurate predictor of the disease status of a pup (encoded at locus **B**) than would marker **C**.

This reasoning is the basis for using molecular markers as diagnostic tests to predict whether or not a particular pup has inherited a gene that will eventually result in its developing the genetic disease. *Obviously, the closer a marker is to the disease gene and the more informative the marker, the more accurate the predictions that can be made.*

## Measuring the accuracy of the linkage

The second basic feature of linkage analysis is a **lod score**. A lod score is a measure of the confidence one can put into a predicted genetic distance between two loci, such as the distance between marker A and the disease gene locus B in figure 12. A large lod score associated with a particular genetic distance means that it is a strong prediction; a small lod score, that it is weaker.

In general, a lod score of 3, corresponding to 1,000 to 1 odds (upper green band of figure 13), is accepted as significant evidence that two loci are located close together or **linked**. Conversely, a lod score of less than minus 2 (lower green band) is accepted as evidence against linkage of the two loci. The middle ground (cream color band) between these scores is ambiguous, and more information would be necessary to either prove or refute linkage between the loci.

The lod score of 6.0 associated with a genetic distance (recombination fraction) of 23 cM between a marker locus A and a disease locus B is very strong support in favor of linkage at a close genetic distance. Marker A would be a reasonable indicator of whether or not a puppy would have inherited from its parent an allele that is involved in disease. Depending on how polymorphic the loci are and other factors, linkage can usually be detected between two loci that are less than 40 cM apart or that are separated by less than 40% recombination. When we can detect linkage between two loci, we also know that they are on the same chromosome, although the converse is not true.

A lod or log of the odds in favor of linkage between two loci is expressed as a log so lod scores for different families that have the same disease, can be calculated separately for each family and then added together.

Making separate calculations for each family is important because disease in all families may not result from mutations or defects in the same gene locus, and pooling results from families with different mutations would obscure the detection of a linkage. Adding the lods together only for families with linkage will strengthen the results.

*linked;* two loci that will be inherited together in the population a high percentage of the time, as evidenced by the calculation of a lod score of 3 or higher.

*lod;* abbreviation for the log of the odds *supporting linkage of two loci, with a score of 3 ($10^3$ or 1,000:1) traditionally accepted as evidence of linkage between two markers or between a marker and a disease gene.*

# *Figure 13. Lod scores chart the likelihood of linkage.*

The odds that a marker is linked to a hypothetical disease gene can be expressed as a lod score and shown as a graph. In this example the lod score is 6, which is the equivalent of 1,000,000 to 1 odds in favor of linkage (also expressed as $10^6$ odds), with a genetic distance of approximately 23 cM (or a recombination fraction of .23) between the marker and disease gene (arrow on horizontal scale highlighted by the blue dog).

The upper green band of the graph (red arrow "evidence in favor of linkage") corresponds to greater than 1,000 to 1 odds

in favor of linkage, or a lod score of 3, which is the level traditionally accepted as the threshold above which a linkage is considered to be present.

This figure is a graphed representation of the events depicted in figure 12 between loci A and B if the lod score associated with the distance between loci A and B is 6.0. This means that the odds for the distance of 23 cM between A and B is $10^6$ or 1,000,000 to 1 that this is the correct distance. We can be quite confident the markers (or marker A and disease gene B) are linked at a distance between them of 23 cM.

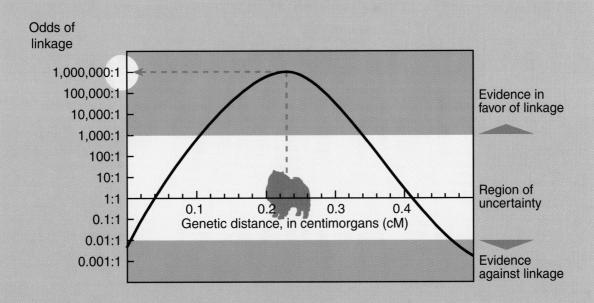

## To test your understanding . . .

Figure 13 shows a plot of data for a marker that is 23 cM from a disease gene (arrow) and also has a lod score of 6.0 ($10^6$ or 1,000,000:1). What would the plot for marker A and disease gene B look like if they were much closer, say only 1 cM ($\theta = 0.01$) apart with a lod score of 10? The peak for linkage between A and B would be midway between the first tick mark on the horizontal scale, and the peak in figure 13 would be off the verticle scale (up to 10,000,000,000 or 10 billion to 1 odds).

Would this marker be a better predictor of disease inheritance in the pups than the one shown in figure 13? Yes, because the marker is closer to the disease gene and so less likely to be separated from it by a recombination event. Also, the lod score is much higher, increasing our confidence in the prediction.

If the peak between B and C was greater than 0.5 (off the horizontal scale), what would it look like? The height was not given and so could not be plotted without more information, but it would be unlinked at 50 cM.

---

A lod score is calculated as the probability of a particular distance between two loci (A and B in the example) that varies by computer iteration, divided by the distance at which no linkage can be detected between two loci, (recombination fraction of 0.5 or $\theta = 0.5$). While this explanation sounds complicated, the formula for the calculation it describes is actually simple.

While the formula may be simple, the process of calculating a lod score requires considerable computational effort to find the maximum likelihood value. Relatively recent modifications of the formula to improve accuracy have made the calculations even more time consuming. The calculations are so computationally intensive that for practical purposes they could not even be done until 1985, when relatively high-speed computers became more widely available.

It is certainly not necessary to understand how genetic distances and their associated confidence measures (lod scores) are calculated to understand how they are used in the prediction of risk for inherited disease. A basic understanding of these concepts aids in understanding the use and reliability of a genetic test for predicting disease risk.

---

Those who would like to understand linkage analysis in greater detail can refer to the excellent text, *Handbook of Human Linkage Analysis* by Terwilliger and Ott (1994), The Johns Hopkins Press.

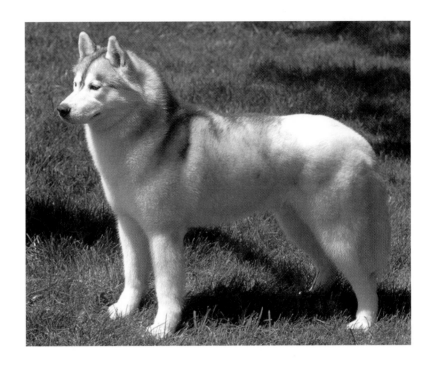

*The Siberian Husky was originally bred by the Chukchi people of northeastern Asia. It was imported to North America in large numbers after 1910 for racing over the rugged Alaskan terrain. The Husky is friendly, gentle and independent, but retains its natural desire to roam.*

## Determining the inheritance of favorable traits

Identical methods can be used to determine the inheritance of favorable traits or characteristics, if they can be reliably detected and have one of the simple modes of inheritance. To carry out this analysis, one would need to know the trait status of each pedigree member instead of the disease status. The linkage analysis and interpretation of the results is identical, whether seeking a marker for a disease gene or a gene specifying a desirable trait or characteristic.

A physical map, by comparison to a genetic map created by linkage analysis, gives information about the *actual* chromosomal location and relative order of markers, *without* information about the distance between loci. A physical map is created by hybridization of a piece of DNA containing a marker locus to a chromosome spread much like that made to produce the beginning of the karyotype seen in figure 3a on page 15.

### Combining genetic maps and physical maps

It is very useful to integrate maps made with the two different methods by mapping some markers both ways. This comparison confirms the marker order, identifies the chromosomal location for a set of markers that are connected by linkage analysis and identifies areas between linked groups of markers that are too far apart to be linked together using linkage analysis.

"Holes" in the genetic map may be filled by adding new markers to the map. As more markers are added, it is generally possible to produce a map of linked markers that covers each chromosome.

*The Cocker Spaniel may have been named for its superior ability to hunt woodcock. It is a capable gun dog which can be trained to flush and retrieve game from both land and water. It is also a playful companion.*

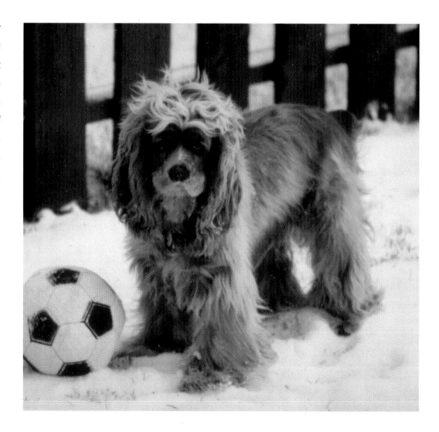

# Selecting the best genes: key to the future

## Finding flanking markers improves the accuracy of prediction

When trait and disease genes are located on a map of high marker density (markers every 5–10 cM), it is immediately evident which markers flank the gene, and its location can be more precisely identified using many markers to position it. **Multipoint linkage analysis** places the gene of interest in the most likely position on a marker map of known order and distance. By adding markers to increase the density of the map, markers closer and closer to the gene of interest will be identified.

*The direct usefulness of these techniques then begins to become apparent to dog breeders.* Markers close to a disease gene are very important for an accurate diagnostic test. The closer a marker is to a disease gene, the better predictor the test will be. Although a diagnostic test can be done with only one linked marker, a test using two linked markers that flank the disease gene is far more accurate.

## A direct diagnostic test

Eventually, after markers very close to the gene are found (usually within 1–2 cM), it becomes possible to actually isolate and clone the disease gene, to determine the sequence of its DNA bases.

When the sequence of a disease gene is known, it can be compared to the normal gene sequence and the mutation identified, as has already been done for several human diseases. From this information, a **direct diagnostic test** can be developed. Identification of specific gene mutations makes the more accurate direct diagnostic test possible, and enables further studies to determine how the mutant gene produces the observable disease symptoms.

*multipoint linkage analysis;* the use of a map segment composed of multiple markers to more precisely place a gene of interest relative to the known map.

*direct diagnostic test;* a test that is based on examining the actual region of a possible gene defect to predict the inheritance of a disease.

For some human diseases, work has already progressed to this point, and many ingenious methods are being attempted to modify or stop the disease process. Disease genes and normal genes involved in relavant biological processes that have been identified in other organisms — usually humans or laboratory mice — can also be tested as **candidate genes** for canine diseases. With luck and careful guesswork, sometimes a shortcut to a direct test can be discovered this way (for example, the test for vWD in Manchester Terriers, Shelties, Dobermans, Poodles, Pembroke Welsh Corgis, and Scotties). In the past, direct tests have also been developed for diseases where a structural protein or enzyme, or other functional defect is known.

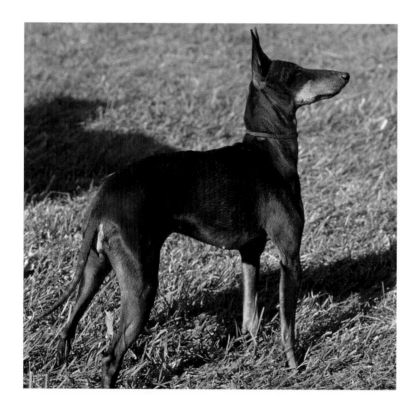

*The graceful and sleek Manchester Terrier is thought to be derived from a dark brown rat-killing terrier crossed with a Whippet, Italian Greyhound, Greyhound, and possibly the early Dachshund. Its skills include rabbit coursing.*

Every advance provides new information and an improved ability to deal with an inherited disease. From the first relatively crude diagnostic test done with only one marker, to the increasingly improved diagnostic tests that become possible as the flanking markers are placed closer and closer to the disease gene, each discovery moves closer to the direct test, with its more certain answers.

## Marker-assisted selection: the key to eliminating disorders, salvaging desirable characteristics

Every breeder's attempt to produce quality purebred dogs includes a strong commitment to reduce inherited disease in their breed. Line-breeding, the tool largely responsible for creating the tremendous variety of dog breeds we know today, also aggregates deleterious genes to produce recessive and polygenic disorders.

### Recessive traits and genetic testing

Recessive and polygenic disorders are insidious, going undetected until the condition becomes frequent enough to be recognized as inherited. Generations may be unaffected when carriers are rare. However, in time, unaffected carriers become common. With linebreeding, more affected individuals will appear in a breed unless unaffected carriers can be identified and selective breeding practiced.

Removing affected individuals from the breeding population still leaves many carriers. With a recessive trait, all offspring of affected individuals, two-thirds of their normal full-siblings, half of any offspring of each parent and half the full-siblings of both parents would carry a deleterious allele and yet appear normal (figure 6b). Until recently available molecular diagnostic methods began to be used, there was little chance of eliminating all carriers from a breeding program, because they could not be identified until affected offspring were produced. With late onset diseases, disease status often would not be known until many litters were produced.

### Dominant diseases and genetic testing

Without appropriate genetic tests, the picture for autosomal dominant diseases is not appreciably better. In diseases that show early symptoms clear enough for diagnosis, affected dogs can be removed from the breeding population. This action decreases the prevalence of the deleterious allele. However, dogs inheriting a disease allele and their owners are not spared the consequences of the inherited disease.

**candidate gene;** a gene that results in a similar disease in another organism or that is thought to be biologically relevant to the canine disease through comparison to other organisms.

**marker assisted selection;** the use of genetic markers for selection of a linked desirable characteristic or trait, or against a disease gene.

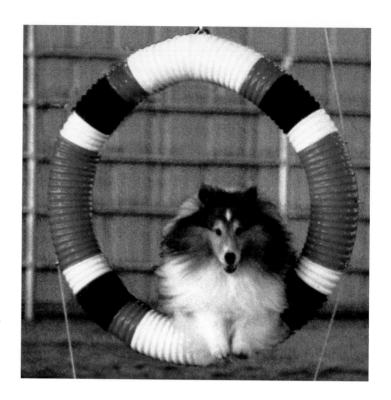

*The sensitivity and responsiveness of the Shetland Sheepdog allows them to be easily trained and makes them excellent companions and watchdogs.*

In early onset diseases with variable severity of symptoms, mild cases often go unrecognized until a severely affected puppy is produced and the gene has already been spread in the population. In dominant diseases in which symptoms are not apparent until post-breeding age, little can be done to stop the spread. In such cases, half of the progeny produced by a parent bearing the disease gene are destined to become affected, as will the parents themselves, eventually, if they live long enough to show the symptoms.

Now, with the development of genetic tests for a few dominantly and recessively inherited disorders, breeders can identify at an early age dogs that are likely to pass on these disease genes. In this way breeding programs can be modified by testing before breeding. The result will be genetically healthier dogs in these breeds. However, we have barely begun to reap the possible benefits from this technology and there are still numerous inherited diseases in many breeds for which we need to develop diagnostic tests. Those few tests already developed are significant illustrations of what can be done in the future to eliminate the inherited diseases found in many more breeds.

It is already clear that *when diagnostic tests are available and used wisely, it is far easier for breeders to concentrate desirable characteristics, and to produce healthier and better quality dogs.* An inherited disease gene becomes just another characteristic to be taken into consideration when arranging a breeding or deciding which pups are of sufficient quality to consider as possible breeding stock. It does not become the dreaded specter that might end a show career, relegate an active performance dog to the couch, or worst of all, make euthanasia a benevolent release for a beloved pet.

## Clinical and husbandry benefits of genetic testing

There are other incentives to use presymptomatic tests to detect inherited disorders:

1.  The genetic test information will allow breeders to move toward their goals more rapidly without the set-backs of unexpected inherited diseases in their breeding stock.

2.  Genetic test information aids veterinarians in differential diagnosis, facilitating earlier treatment before disease weakens the dog seriously and allowing for more effective disease management.

3.  Veterinarians can use information gained from presymptomatic diagnostic tests to minimize late-appearing symptoms, in those diseases in which early medical or surgical intervention influences disease severity.

Clearly, from all perspectives, there is little to lose and an enormous amount to be gained in the use of genetic tests that detect inherited diseases.

We have years of work ahead using the available methods to reduce the multitude of inherited diseases that have simple (dominant, recessive and sex-linked) modes of inheritance. As we attempt to go beyond the mapping of traits and diseases with simple modes of inheritance to those due to the action of multiple genes, it will become necessary to develop maps of markers tailored to be maximally informative in each breed under study.

*informative marker;*
*a marker with many alleles of relatively even frequency distribution; this can vary by breed and even line and family within a breed, depending on the marker.*

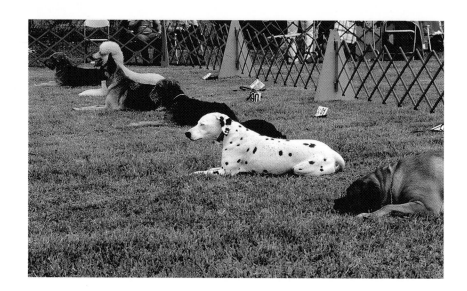

*The "long down" exercise demonstrates that a variety of breeds can compete effectively in obedience events. A single marker would not be equally informative and therefore useful for mapping an inherited disease in each of these different breeds. Consequently, it is necessary to select the markers that are most useful for each breed.*

## Marker informativeness differs by breed

Marker-assisted selection is the use of one or more markers that are linked to any trait or characteristic of interest, whether a disease or desirable gene, to aid in deciding which animals will be most useful in improving the next generation of offspring. The most informative marker is highly polymorphic in the breed population, and the closer it is to the trait of interest, the more accurate a prediction it permits.

When a mated pair has four different alleles at a locus, in the offspring it is unambiguous which allele is inherited from each parent. Thus, the marker is maximally informative in this instance. Where there is a high probability of this situation occuring many times in a breed population, the marker is highly informative *in that breed.*

Early research shows that all markers are not equally polymorphic, hence, not equally informative in all dog breeds. Since breeders have selected for tremendous variety while producing the various dog breeds, they also have been selecting for different degrees of polymorphism in linked microsatellite markers. Thus, it is useful to sort out which markers are most polymorphic in each breed. To do this, representative samples of DNA from unrelated dogs of each breed are collected and markers genotyped. Identifying the set of markers that is most informative in each breed (a breed-informative set or **BISmarkers**™) and assembling them into a genetic map yields a **BISmap**™.

**BISmaps**™ will be essential for mapping diseases and traits in each particular breed, particularly complex traits. It may be necessary to use different markers for diagnostic linkage tests developed for use in different breeds. This could be true even if diseases the markers detect are due to mutations in the same gene. It will also be more likely to be necessary initially, when a disease-linked marker is located at a greater distance from the gene of interest. As closer markers are identified, the same markers are more likely to be informative in different breeds, if the disease is due to the same mutation in a common distant ancestor. Alternatively, several different mutations of a particular gene may result in a disease found in several dog breeds (i.e., the mutations arose independently in different dog breeds affected with a disease that appears similar clinically).

Studies of human disease confirm that it is also possible for mutations in different genes to produce the same clinical picture. This is not surprising when we consider that such genes can encode mutant proteins that act in different successive steps of a pathway or in pathways that merge to produce a final common product. The bottom line is that it does not matter how a defect is produced; if the final product cannot do its normal job, the clinical problem will be similar. Diseases that are produced by defects in different genes, but look like a single clinical entity, are called **genetically heterogeneous.**

## Value of familial lod scores

Because of the possibility for genetic heterogeneity, calculating lod scores separately for each family is desirable when attempting to identify markers linked to disease genes. Since lod scores can be added together, even small families can contribute to the overall significance of the lod score. Many small families can be sampled and tested for linkage between the disease and a marker may be found to be linked only in one family, in several families, or in all of the families.

**BISmap**™; the genetic map assembled from BIS markers, creating a maximally informative breed map.

**BISmarkers**™; the "breed informative set" of genetic markers that constitute the most informative markers available for a given breed.

**genetic heterogeneity;** when mutations in different genes produce a clinically similar picture within a breed.

Families that contribute to the lod score can be separated from those that do not, which helps to sort out the situation with respect to genetic heterogeneity. The approach of calculating lod scores separately for each family can also be used when a disease with a similar clinical picture appears in multiple breeds. If the breeds are related somewhere back in their genetic history, similar diseases observed in them may be due to a gene mutation in a common ancestor that has been inherited by individuals that were the progenitors of both breeds. Alternatively, it is also possible that mutations in a gene that confers disease has arisen independently in more than one line or more than one breed.

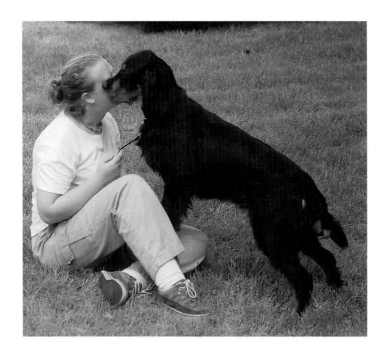

*The Gordon Setter has been known since the 1600s as a methodical, dependable and responsive bird dog. The breed standard allows a range of sizes to accommodate the variety of hunting terrains. It is a loyal and devoted companion and guard dog.*

### Marker assisted selection can work well for dog breeders

When the two alleles are different on each of a dog's two homologous chromosomes (i.e., the dog is heterozygous at this locus), their inheritance can be followed through a pedigree (figure 9a). If the presence or absence of disease in each pedigree member is also known, linkage analysis can determine which allele is traveling with the disease gene in a particular family (figure 9b). A marker allele that is inherited with the disease gene in a particular pedigree is said to **segregate** with the disease gene.

Conversely, the disease phenotype or observable characteristics segregate with the marker genotype. The more tightly linked the marker is to the trait, the more often there will be correspondence between inheritance of a marker allele and the trait in a family.

When a particular marker is known to be linked to a disease gene and parent/offspring genotypes for this locus are known, the genetic distance between the two loci can be used to predict how likely each puppy born to these parents is to be affected by the disease. This is their **risk** of inheriting the disease-producing allele.

In a disease with a dominant mode of inheritance, puppies inheriting the same marker allele as the affected parent will have a risk for inheriting the disease that is proportional to the distance between the marker and the disease gene. If the marker is very close (for example, if marker A and disease gene B in figure 12 were 1 cM apart), puppies inheriting a marker allele from an affected parent are highly likely to inherit the disease gene. Inheritance with the other parental allele is less likely because the occurrence of a recombination event causing the disease gene to be inherited with it would be very rare.

## Accuracy of linkage and direct tests

It is, of course, possible that a recombination event might occur and make prediction about the disease status of a particular puppy wrong. We would expect a diagnostic test based on a marker mapped 1 cM away from the disease gene to be wrong an average of 1 percent of the time. In this case, a recombination event will *prevent* the puppy from inheriting the disease gene 1% of the time. For this reason, a diagnostic test based on linkage analysis can not be accurate 100% of the time. Only a diagnostic test based on actually examining for the disease gene mutation (sometimes called a **direct test**) has the potential to be accurate all of the time.

*direct test;* a diagnostic test based on examining for the presence of the actual disease-producing genetic mutation.

*risk;* the probability that offspring of a particular mating will be affected by a disease; risk of disease inheritance can be predicted when the genetic distance between a marker and a disease-causing gene is known along with the individual's genotype.

*segregate;* when a marker is inherited together with a disease or desirable gene in a particular pedigree.

### Breeder use of genetic tests

Despite these frustrating caveats, using biotechnology to accurately predict disease is a significant improvement over the alternative. For a disease with an **autosomal dominant** mode of inheritance, on average, 50% of the puppies produced by an affected dog will be affected, but without a diagnostic test, we have no idea which ones will be until they show signs. Once a diagnostic test is available, puppies can be tested at birth or before they are placed. Cord blood from the pup's placenta or samples collected at dew claw removal, tail docking or ear cropping time would be adequate for testing. Some laboratories even routinely isolate genomic DNA and perform diagnostic tests out of a brushing taken from the inside of the cheek.

Puppies destined to be affected with an inherited disease, even diseases that don't become apparent until well past reproductive age, can be immediately identified as poor candidates for breeding. If the disease in question strikes early and has a poor prognosis for even a short lifetime of reasonable quality, the breeder might elect to spare the puppy trauma and euthanize it.

If the disease in question were incompletely penetrant or had a late onset, the breeder would probably plan not to use the puppy for breeding as an adult, since 50% of its offspring would again inherit the disease gene, but the puppy might have a fair chance at a reasonable quality life. The 50% of puppies in the litter that were determined by the diagnostic test *not to have inherited the disease gene* could safely be used for breeding, if their other qualities warrant it. Used wisely and over successive generations, molecular diagnostic tests can rapidly eliminate undesirable genes from a breed gene pool.

Using linked molecular markers to detect a disease transmitted with a **recessive** mode of inheritance is even more advantageous than for a dominantly inherited disease. Puppies that carry only one gene for the disease will pass this allele on to half their offspring but will never have the disease themselves. This is because a recessive mode of inheritance requires two disease alleles at the disease locus for expression of the disorder. Therefore, a dog with the disease will always be a homozygote at the disease locus (as was seen with the middle dog of the litter of five, alleles 177/177, in figure 9b on page 47).

**autosomal dominant disease;** when inheritance of only one mutant allele results in a disease.

**recessive disease;** when two similar mutant alleles at a locus are required to produce a disease.

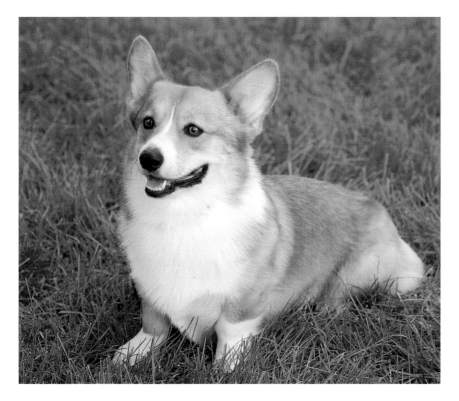

*The Corgi is one of several breeds with inherited von Willebrand's disease (vWD) or blood clotting Factor VIII anomaly. The mode of inheritance in some breeds is dominant and in others recessive. There are also several types that are due to different mutations. A direct test is available for detecting carriers and presymptomatic affected dogs in several breeds including the Pembroke Welsh Corgi. A test developed for use in one breed may shorten development of similar tests for other breeds.*

Without a molecular diagnostic test for a recessive disease, a carrier can be identified only by producing an affected pup. Since this requires breeding two carriers, when the disease is rare in the population, it may take many breedings before this happens by chance. Meanwhile, the carrier passes on the disease gene to half of all offspring, spreading it throughout the breeding population. As the disease gene becomes more common, more affected puppies are produced.

The inadvertant spread of a recessive disorder can and has happened before breeders have recognized that a particular disease was inherited, and not due to environmental trauma or infection, etc.

A diagnostic test for a recessive inherited disease can rapidly change this situation. By testing the prospective sire and dam prior to breeding, *an affected puppy need never be produced* except by error in prediction, which should become increasingly rare as discovery of markers closer and closer to the disease gene produce more accurate diagnostic tests.

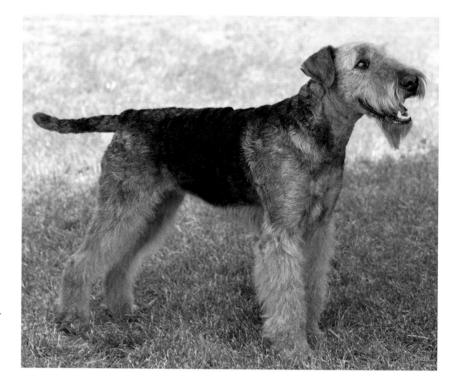

*The Airedale Terrier is one of many breeds with a higher than average risk (genetic predisposition) for malignant tumors. Progress in understanding the genetics of human cancers should aid in pinpointing genes involved in the many canine cancers.*

Obviously, *two known carriers should never be mated,* but a known carrier with other significant compelling qualities could be safely mated to a known non-carrier and the puppies tested. No affected puppies would result, and the half of the litter that are carriers could be placed with nonbreeding registration to live out completely healthy and normal lives unless they too had other compelling positive qualities to offer.

In other words, carrier status for an inherited disease could become just another factor (though an important one) in deciding which puppies are of sufficient quality to be used for breeding. This is true if *a breeder is willing to go to the extra expense of having the prospective mate of a carrier and all puppies produced tested for carrier status.* However, it must be remembered that if carriers are not reduced in the breed population by conscientious breeders, the disease gene will spread, and *eventually, the choice of non-carrier mates for disease carriers will become limited.*

## Implications for rare breeds

In rare breeds, it is *not desirable to eliminate all of the carriers of a particular disease immediately*. This is because of the risk of decreasing the genetic variability of the breed to an unhealthy level. Molecular diagnostic tests are most effectively used in small breed populations to avoid producing affected dogs while maintaining the genetic variability by continuing to breed superior carriers and unaffected dogs.

Reducing genetic variation by using molecular diagnostic tests is less likely to be a problem in a common breed with a large breeding population, particularly when carriers are still relatively rare in the breed. When carriers are common in a popular breed, the breeding population should be managed much like a rare breed by continuing to breed carriers but to avoid producing affected dogs.

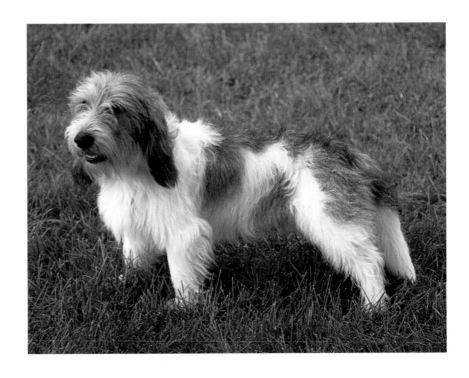

*Petit Basset Griffon Vendeen, a rabbit hunter developed in France to hunt game over densely vegetated terrain, is still a relatively rare breed in the U.S. It became eligible to compete in AKC sponsored events in 1991.*

## Diagnostic tests for traits with a polygenic mode of inheritance

A disease or desirable trait that has a polygenic mode of inheritance can also be mapped. It does, however, require considerably more work. The methods used for producing genotypes (**genotyping**) are the same, but the data analysis is somewhat different.

The analysis for polygenic inheritance requires a genomic map of markers spaced at approximately 40 cM intervals. A family (usually covering three generations) that has been characterized for the trait of interest, is genotyped with the markers, and the interval between each set of two markers is examined to see if the trait inheritance correlates. This is done using a statistical method of analysis called least squares regression.

### "Where do I get the tests?"

Development of diagnostic genetic tests is proceeding rapidly, and printed lists fall quickly out of date. Tests available as of the date this copy of *FutureDog* was initially distributed are noted on an information card in a pocket on the inside of the back cover.

Information on this update card was current as of the date of release noted on it. For more current information, contact the AKC Canine Health Foundation, or check their World Wide Web site at:

**www.akcchf.org**

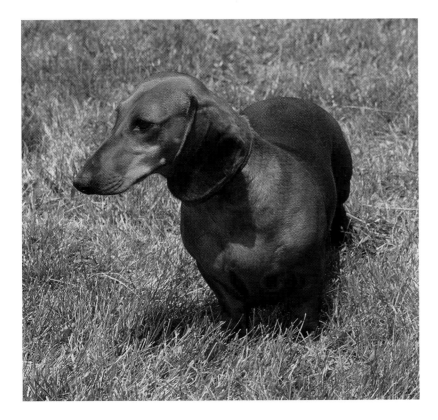

*The Dachshund or, literally, "badger dog" required strength, stamina and courage for the hunt of boar, rabbit and fox. Today's Dachshunds are hardy, playful companions and watchdogs, in either standard or miniature size, with three coat varieties and many color variations.*

Where a relatively small number of genes contribute to the disease phenotype, it has been possible to identify them in at least one human disease. This method, sometimes called **interval analysis**, is currently being used to identify the genes contributing to traits of economic importance in several livestock species.

## Some molecular diagnostic tests are already available

Diagnostic tests for several diseases are already available commercially for a limited number of dog breeds. A great deal of work remains to be done to provide diagnostic tests for many more inherited diseases in more dog breeds.

**genotyping;** *determining the alleles present at a particular locus on an individual's DNA.*

**interval analysis;** *a statistical technique used to locate genes that contribute to traits with polygenic inheritance patterns by examining the intervals between mapped markers for evidence of a gene contributing to the characteristic of interest.*

**polygenic;** *a complex inheritance pattern that can be thought of as a group of genes acting together to produce a particular phenotype.*

### *First steps to early detection of genetic diseases: observation, record keeping, communication*

*One of the most important things that needs to be done can be done by observant breeders and breed clubs.* Breeders can help identify inherited diseases by keeping careful records of any abnormalities they observe.

Once breeders have assembled a record of abnormalities they suspect are genetic, they should then discuss their observations with a knowledgable veterinarian to see if there is any evidence for inheritance of the disease. If what might be an inherited abnormality is seen in several generations of dogs or in related lines, make other breeders aware of them, so that they can watch for similar problems and keep accurate records of their affected dogs.

*The Newfoundland is best known for its water rescue skills. It is also a capable carting dog and has been used to carry heavy packs. Though physically massive and muscular, it is a gentle playmate and nursemaid for children.*

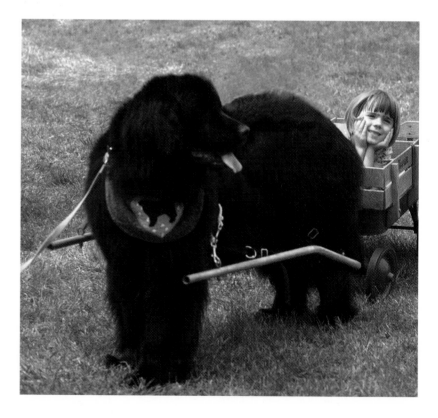

### *First step in genetic research: determine the mode of inheritance*

The next important thing that can be done is to determine the mode of inheritance of a familial disease. Working together, breed clubs and researchers interested in the problem can begin to develop a diagnostic test for the disorder. A clinically recognizable disease with a known mode of inheritance will be the one that researchers are the most interested in working on. This is particularly true if good records have been kept and a breed club has a network of cooperative breeders willing to help by providing samples and pedigree information.

The incentive for breeders is that as diagnostic tests are developed, those who have provided samples from their dogs will be the first to have predictive information about risk of disease inheritance in their puppies.

Once a diagnostic test is available, breed clubs can assist their members and their breeders by seeing that it is used wisely. Affected and carrier dogs can be sold with contracts that clearly stipulate the buyer's obligations with regard to breeding.

*It is no disgrace to breed a dog with an inherited disorder accidentally and unknowingly.* Remember, the gene was almost certainly already in the breed population before a particular breeding was decided upon. The best a breeder can do in this situation is to make it less likely to happen again by making others aware of potential problems, and by seeking to eliminate the gene that produces the disorder from the line and eventually from the breed. The sooner an inherited disorder is detected in the breed population, the sooner it can be eliminated by the rapid development of a diagnostic test to help the breeder identify both carriers and those destined to become affected.

Because dog breeders rely on linebreeding for progress in shaping the desirable attributes of breeds, they will inadvertently also bring the mutant genes together that result in inherited recessive and polygenic diseases. The dogs that suffer from these disorders can do nothing to stop their spread. Only conscientious breeders and owners of purebred dogs can help save future generations from being afflicted.

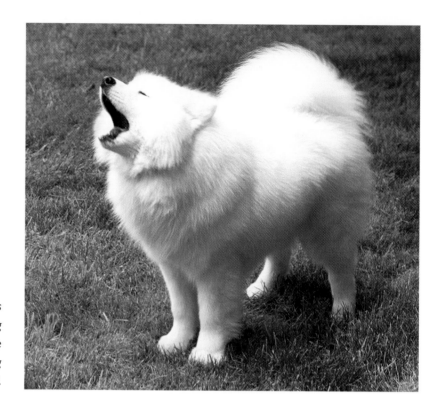

*The vocal Samoyed reminds us that communication among breeders and researchers is the key to effectively combating inherited diseases in every breed.*

## Breeders are the key

**The breeder is the first line of awareness.** Breeders who raise a flag to help others, help themselves and the breed they cherish at the same time. Dog breeders are "in this together" whether they like it or not, because the ancestors of a breed are all related to some degree or another. The only recourse in dealing with inherited diseases is careful observation and conscientious breeding. Now, with the tools that are becoming available, the informed breeders have more options and more solutions to problems than ever before. *In addition, breeders are in the unique position of being able to increase the rate of progress made toward development of useful diagnostic tests by entering into productive and mutually cooperative collaborations with researchers.*

# *Glossary*

**alleles;** the exact same or slightly different alternative forms of a gene, one inherited from each parent.

**amplified;** copying of a section of DNA chemically billions of times.

**anticipation;** earlier and earlier onset in successive generations afflicted with an inherited disease.

**autosomal dominant disease;** when inheritance of only one mutant allele on any non-X or non-Y chromosome results in a disease.

**BISmap™;** the genetic map assembled from BISmarkers™, creating a map that is maximally informative in a particular breed.

**BISmarkers™;** the "breed informative set" of genetic markers that constitute the most informative markers available for a given breed.

**breed;** a group of genetically related dogs with specific characteristics that are readily recognizable, are maintained by selective breeding, and can be predictably anticipated from the matings of appropriate breeding pairs.

**candidate gene;** a gene that results in a similar disease in another organism or that is thought to be biologically relevant to the canine disease through comparison to other organisms.

**centiMorgan (cM);** closely related to a "recombination fraction," a measurement of the genetic distance between a pair of loci which tells us how likely it is that they will be inherited together on a single piece of nonrecombinant DNA.

**chromatid;** two identical copies of a chromosome replicated during meiosis, each eventually becoming a new chromosome as new cells form.

**deoxyribonucleic acid (DNA);** the genetic material of living organisms, transmitted from generation to generation, which specifies the characteristics an offspring inherits from its parents.

**direct diagnostic test;** a diagnostic test that is based on examining for the presence of the actual disease-producing genetic mutations to predict the inheritance of a disease.

**dominant;** when the presence of only one copy of a particular gene results in the inheritance of an observable trait or disease.

**DNA profile;** also known as a "DNA fingerprint;" a composite of a set of approximately a dozen highly polymorphic genetic markers that characterizes the individual uniquely.

**electrophoresis;** a process used to sort PCR-amplified DNA fragments into bands that make up an individual genotype for a particular locus; where fragments of amplified DNA migrate through a gel matrix, sorted by size into bands.

**epistatic effect;** when genes at one locus influence the expression of genes at another locus.

**gametes;** the male's sperm cells and the female's eggs (ova).

**genes;** the biochemical sequences of DNA that constitute the functional units of heredity that are transmitted from generation to generation, and which are ultimately translated into proteins that carry out specific structural or enzymatic functions.

**genetic heterogeneity;** when mutations in different genes produce a clinically similar picture within a breed; can happen where different mutations affect different genes that act sequentially in a single pathway, where a defect anywhere in the pathway may produce the same end result or disease symptoms.

**genetic map;** a map showing the location of genetic markers relative to each other and genetic distances between markers.

**genomic DNA;** DNA that includes more than the biologically meaningful segments that encode genes; it includes sequences of regulatory DNA as well as DNA with no known function.

**genotype;** the genetic constitution of an individual that is characterized by a marker or a banding pattern at a particular locus.

**genotyping;** determining the alleles present at a particular locus on an individual's DNA.

**heterozygote;** where two alleles that are slightly different in their nucleotide sequences are present at a particular locus on the respective chromosomes of a homologous pair.

**homozygote;** where two identical alleles are present on the respective chromosomes of a homologous pair.

**homologous;** a pair of chromosomes that are similar in size and shape, and encode the same genes in the same order but may vary slightly in sequence of DNA.

**inbreeding;** matings between closely related dogs, such as between first degree relatives (to parent, sibling, or its own offspring).

**incompletely penetrant;** when a particular gene is inherited but the phenotype expected is not expressed (observed).

**independent assortment;** the random distribution of chromosomes, during meiosis, to what eventually become egg and sperm cells.

**informative;** a marker that provides the maximum amount of inheritance information possible.

**informative marker;** a marker with many alleles of relatively even frequency distribution; this can vary by breed and even line and family within a breed, depending on the marker.

**interval analysis;** a statistical technique used to locate genes that contribute to traits with polygenic inheritance patterns by examining the intervals between mapped markers for evidence of a gene contributing to the characteristic of interest.

**karyotype;** pairs of homologous chromosomes that are aligned by similar size, shape and banding pattern.

**linebreeding;** a breeding between dogs with a common ancestor, but one that is more distantly related than with inbreeding.

**linkage analysis;** a method invented in the early 1900s for estimating the genetic distances between loci.

**linked;** two loci that will be inherited together in the population a high percentage of the time, as evidenced by the calculation of a lod score of 3 or higher; usually detectable if they are less than 40 cM apart.

**locus;** the location of a gene or microsatallite marker sequence.

**lod;** abbreviation for the *log of the odds* supporting linkage of two loci, with a score of 3 ($10^3$ or 1,000:1) traditionally accepted as evidence of linkage between two markers or between a marker and a disease gene.

**lod score;** the *log of the odds* supporting linkage of two loci, with a score of 3 traditionally accepted as evidence of linkage between two markers or between a marker and a disease gene.

**marker;** a reliable identifier of the same specific and unique location on genomic DNA.

**marker assisted selection;** the use of genetic markers for selection of a linked desirable characteristic or trait, or against a disease gene.

**meiosis;** the production of individual gametes (an egg or sperm cells) through doubling, recombination and then reduction of genetic material.

**Mendelian inheritance;** the pattern of gene inheritance originally described by Gregor Mendel; the inheritance of one copy of a gene (allele) from each parent by its offspring.

**microsatellite markers;** short tandem repeats of nucleotide sequences also known as short tandem repeat polymorphisms (STRP) that are flanked by unique sequence PCR primers and are used to examine inherited polymorphisms.

**monomorphic;** no observable variation at a particular locus, i.e. it has only one possible form or allele present in a population.

**morphological;** pertaining to the morphology or observable physical form of a particular trait or characteristic.

**multipoint linkage analysis;** the use of a map segment composed of multiple markers to more precisely place a gene of interest relative to the known map.

**mutation;** a biological mistake that introduces variation into a genome which can be harmful, favorable or have no apparent effect.

**oligonucleotide primers;** small stretches of unique sequence DNA selected to flank a tandem repeat sequence that are used as primers for amplifying the segment of DNA contained between them.

**phenotype;** the appearance or behavior of a breed or individual that can be directly observed.

**polygenic;** a complex inheritance pattern that can be thought of as a group of genes acting together to produce a particular phenotype.

**polymerase chain reaction (PCR);** the process used to amplify a segment of DNA to provide billions of copies.

**polymorphic;** when more than one possible allele exists at a locus within a breed population.

**polymorphism;** the variation between a particular gene and its mate on a pair of homologous chromosomes.

**recessive;** two identical alleles at a locus producing a particular characteristic, trait or disease.

**recessive disease;** when two similar mutant alleles at a locus are required to produce a disease.

**recombination;** physical breakage and reunion of DNA strands that results in genetic variation.

**replicate;** when a chromosome is duplicated during meiosis.

**risk;** the probability that offspring of a particular mating will be affected by a disease; risk of disease inheritance can be predicted when the genetic distance between a marker and a disease-causing gene is known along with the individual's genotype.

**segregate;** when a marker is inherited together with a disease or desirable gene in a particular pedigree.

**selective breeding;** deliberate choice of mating pairs, with the retention of offspring having desirable traits for future breedings.

**synapse, synapsis;** joining of homologous chromosomes in the regions where they are similar that occurs just prior to recombination.

**type;** the sum total of characteristics and traits that typify a particular breed and are essential to making it distinctive from other breeds or lineages within a breed.

# Suggested reading

*This is a brief annotated list for readers interested in learning more about animal genetics and biotechnology. Some volumes on this list are available through booksellers or their publishers. Others are currently out of print but should be readily available through public libraries or inter-library loan services.*

**Animals by Design: A Primer on the Tools of Modern Biotechnology** (1998) Minnesota Agricultural Experiment Station, University of Minnesota, St. Paul, Minnesota, 28 pages. This is a brief discussion of how the tools of biotechnology are applied to select for traits of economic importance in agricultural livestock. It is written for a non-technical reader.

**Control of Canine Genetic Diseases** (1998) George A. Padget, Howell Book House, New York, New York, 264 pages. ISBN 0-87605-004-6. Offers practical information and advice on inherited canine diseases for breeders, including many question and answer sets to test understanding of the concepts.

**Genetics for Dog Breeders** (1990) Roy Robinson, Pergamon Press, Inc., Elmsford, New York, 280 pages. ISBN 0-08-037492-1. This book includes a discussion of many of the inherited diseases affecting dogs, as well as sections on basic genetics and reproduction.

**Genetics of the Dog** (1989) Malcolm B. Willis, Howell Book House, New York, New York, 416 pages. ISBN 0-87605-551-X. This book offers clear well-illustrated explanations of basic and population genetics discussed with reference to the dog.

**Handbook of Human Linkage Analysis** (1994) Joseph D. Terwilliger and Jurg Ott, The Johns Hopkins Press, Baltimore, Maryland, 307 pages, ISBN 0-8018-4803-2. With the companion volume authored by Jurg Ott, the definitive information detailing linkage analysis is comprehensively covered from theory to examples. Most of the discussion applies directly to dogs as well as humans. However, these books probably will be of interest only to those with a significant background in statistics.

**Introduction to Veterinary Genetics** (1996) Frank W. Nicholas, Oxford University Press, New York, New York, 317 pages, ISBN 019-854292-5. This book provides good explanations and illustrations of basic genetic principles, and touches briefly on many basic concepts in population genetics. It is the only one of the books mentioned here that discusses modern molecular methods, including short sections on microsatellite polymorphisms, mapping of disease genes and marker-assisted selection.

**Practical Genetics for Dog Breeders** (1992) Malcolm B. Willis, H.F. & G. Witherby, Ltd., Suffolk, United Kingdom, 239 pages, ISBN 0-85493-218-6. Unfortunately, this book is currently out of print but may still be obtainable from catalog booksellers that specialize in dog books (for example, 4M Enterprises, Union City, CA, 510-489-8722). It offers an excellent discussion of polygenic inheritance complete with detailed examples, as well as candid discussions of genetic problems that will confront dog breeders, along with sound genetic advice for dealing with many of them. For serious breeders, the book is well worth the extra effort necessary to obtain a copy.

**Medical and Genetic Aspects of Purebred Dogs** (1994) edited by Ross D. Clark, DVM and Joan R. Stainer, Forum Publications, Inc., Fairway, Kansas, 687 pages, ISBN 0-9641609-0-0. This book briefly describes each breed and reviews inherited diseases common to the breed. It is a good starting point for information about inherited diseases with a reference list for additional details.

**The Domestic Dog: Its Evolution, Behaviour and Interactions with People.** (1995) edited by James Serpell, Cambridge University Press, Melbourne, Australia, 268 pages, ISBN 0-521-42537-9. This book offers a fascinating compendium of dog information not often discussed elsewhere. Reading it is guaranteed to change your understanding of and interactions with dogs, no matter what your starting opinions.

# Canine health related services and information resources

*Developments in this field are proceding rapidly, and across the field of biotechnology commercial firms are being regularly bought and merged, and university based testing laboratories and facilities are being established and reorganized. Only a few of the most stable organizations are listed here. The Canine Health Foundation web site (www.akcchf.org) attempts to maintain a more complete and current listing.*

**AKC Canine Health Foundation**, 251 West Garfield Rd., Suite 160, Aurora, OH 44202, Phone: 330-995-0807 (e-mail: akcchf@aol.com). Provides support for research and educational activities relevant to canine health. *(also see Appendix B, beginning on page 98)*

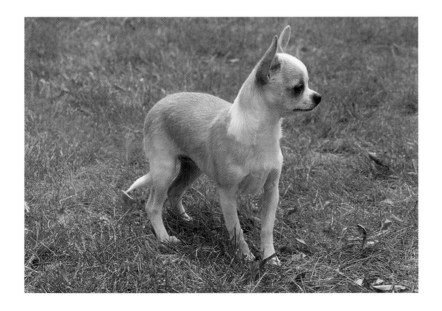

*The Chihuahua, a companion animal often associated with Mexico, was known to exist there more than 500 years ago, during the reign of the Aztec civilization in Central America. It is one of the smallest breeds of dog, with some being as small as two pounds.*

**Canine Eye Registration Foundation (CERF),** SCC-A, Purdue University, W. Lafayette, IN 47907, Phone: 317-494-8179, FAX: 317-494-9981. The Foundation registers eye phenotype evaluations for inherited eye diseases in dogs, provides educational information to the public and maintains a research database.

**Genodermatosis Research Foundation, Inc.,** GRF Secretary, 3838 22nd St. NW, Canton, OH 44708, Phone: 330-478-8322. Provides research support and educational information for inherited skin diseases in several breeds.

**Institute for Genetic Disease Control in Animals (GDC),** P.O. Box 222, Davis, CA 95617, Phone and FAX: 916-756-6773. Maintains open registries for many inherited canine diseases (affected and unaffected individuals are registered) and provides information on testing and diagnosis of these diseases.

**Morris Animal Foundation (MAF),** 45 Inverness Drive East, Englewood, CO 80112-5480, Phone 800-243-2345, FAX 303-790-4066. Supports research on companion and many exotic species.

**Orthopedic Foundation for Animals (OFA),** 2300 Nifong Blvd. Columbia, MO 65201-3856, Phone: 314-442-0418, FAX: 314-875-5073. Maintains a registry of radiographic evaluations, supports research and education with the goal of lowering the incidence of orthopedic and genetic diseases of animals. Registries include hip and elbow dysplasia, patellar luxation, craniomandibular osteopathy, copper toxicosis, thryoid disease and more.

# Appendix A

## Steps to take if you suspect an inherited disorder in your line

1) **Record** and keep updated accurate records of the affected dogs and all related dogs. Even recollections of similar problems in earlier generations may be helpful.

2) **Seek information** and compare information with your veterinarian, other breeders, breed clubs and Parent Breed Clubs, the appropriate registries, etc.

3) If others have seen similar problems, try to determine the **mode of inheritance** of the disorder by examining several generations of dogs in affected pedigrees.

4) Bring the problem to the **attention** of the closest veterinary school, Parent Breed Club health chair, or those doing research on canine inherited disorders. Try to get the problem discussed at local club meetings and the Breed National. If it is widespread in the breed, others will be able to help with steps 1–3. If not, they may become unpleasantly aware of it after an affected or carrier popular sire inadvertently passes the disease gene to many offspring.

# *Appendix B*

## The AKC Canine Health Foundation

### *The Foundation's mission*

The American Kennel Club Canine Health Foundation was established in 1994 to develop programs in basic and applied canine health research and education. The Foundation's primary emphases are improvement of the quality of life for dogs and their owners through the promotion of greater understanding of canine genetics, and development of new diagnostic and therapeutic options for treatment of canine diseases.

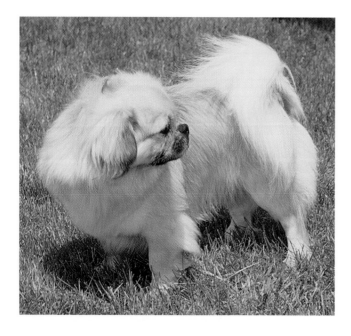

*The Tibetan Spaniel was bred to be a watchdog and is known for its affectionate and trusting personality.*

The Foundation strives to accomplish these goals:

- to help dogs live longer, healthier lives;

- to respect the dedication and interest in canine health of dog clubs, breeders and owners, and to continuously seek ways to involve them in the work of the Foundation;

- to identify health issues of concern to dog owners and breeders;

- to identify and sponsor research and education programs, with particular emphasis on canine genetics, that:

  - meet the highest scientific and educational standards;

  - have the greatest potential for advancing the health of dogs;

  - have expectations for producing materials and applications that are reasonable and affordable.

- to seek ways to integrate the observations and knowledge of dog owners, breeders, veterinarians and other scientists for the purpose of advancing the health of dogs;

- to responsibly monitor grantees and make the results of their work available for public use through publication in scientific journals, and through sharing and dissemination of information and education with dog owners, breeders and veterinarians; and

- to raise endowment funds for the Foundation's programmatic purpose, investing these funds both for growth of the principal and for the generation of income adequate to advance the Foundation's purpose.

The American Kennel Club was founded more than a century ago to promote the study, breeding, exhibiting and advancement of purebred dogs. A strong supporter of canine health research for more than a decade, the AKC pioneered research leading to a vaccine for parvo virus — a deadly killer of puppies and young dogs of all breeds.

The AKC Canine Health Foundation was established as a 501c(3) non-profit organization with the purpose of focusing attention on canine health issues and facilitating research benefiting the health of dogs. As a separate entity, the Foundation is better able to identify and prioritize canine health research objectives, and concentrate the efforts of dog clubs and fanciers working to improve the health of purebred dogs.

In its brief existence, the AKC Canine Health Foundation has become a national and international leader in canine health research. Extraordinary support has come from dog clubs and fanciers, and the scientific community looks to the Foundation as a primary source of funding. The AKC continues to contribute to the Foundation annually to assist in research and administration.

## Support for the highest quality programs

A survey of the 150 AKC Parent Breed Clubs begins the Foundation's grant funding process by identifying the health issues of greatest concern. Then, an annual request for proposal (RFP) is developed, keying on research topics of particular interest. These topics cross four general areas:

- genetics and other conditions specific to particular breeds (for example, cardiomyopathy in Salukis);

- general problems affecting all dogs; such as investigating how long vaccine-induced immunities last;

- basic canine health related research, such as canine genetic and physical mapping;

- advanced canine health education for researchers, dog breeders and veterinarians.

The request for research proposals is widely circulated to veterinary schools, medical schools, research institutions and previous applicants.

## Obtaining funding is very competitive

The Foundation receives more than 100 pre-proposals each year in response to its RFP. Each five-page pre-proposal briefly describes the anticipated project, providing a cost estimate and an outline of the research design. About half of the applicants are subsequently invited to submit a more complete funding application.

Each complete funding application is reviewed by three scientists who are not associated with the proposal's originator or institution. They are evaluated on the research design, facilities available, qualifications of the investigators, and specific relevance to the Foundation's research priorities.

The Foundation does not cover all the expenses involved in a research project. Not funded are overhead or indirect costs, capital equipment costs, salaries of tenured faculty, and travel costs not directly associated with the research. The Foundation funds salaries of post-doctoral staff and laboratory assistants, and supplies and materials related to research projects.

## How you learn what we learn

Each funded research study is separately summarized for lay and for scientific audiences. These abstracts are circulated by the Foundation in a printed "AKC Canine Health Foundation Grants" booklet and are also available online in a searchable data base at the Foundation website (www.akcchf.org).

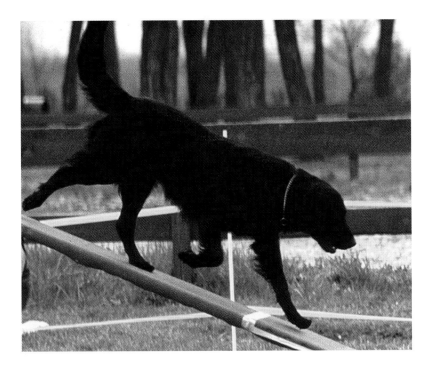

*The Flat-Coated Retriever was developed by selective breeding from the early Newfoundlands, setter, sheepdog and spaniel-like water dogs. The breed retains its natural abilities to hunt and retrieve in thick cover and cold water. Companionable and highly intelligent, it is known for a delightful temperament.*

The Foundation monitors its grantees through semi-annual progress reports for each funded project, reviewed by the Foundation's science officer.

The Foundation encourages scientists to publish results in scientific journals, and itself disseminates the results of sponsored projects by issuing press releases on major findings and by organizing conferences for scientists, Parent Clubs and breeders.

## Fund raising

Raising funds for canine health research and education is a major mission of the Foundation. Donations are accepted from individual dog owners and breeders, and from breed clubs and corporations.

Each year the Foundation asks dog lovers, clubs and corporations to make unrestricted contributions to an annual fund for canine health research. Because the support of the American Kennel Club covers the Foundation's administrative expenses, 100 percent of these annual donations go directly to fund research and educational programs. The annual fund has increased an average of 28 percent per year since it was initiated in 1995.

The Foundation has a Founders Fund recognition program for donors of gifts over $10,000, with a special pin given to recognize individual donors to the fund. Founders Fund contributors are also recognized in special Foundation publications and in each edition of the Canine Health Foundation annual report.

Matching funds for specific approved research are also provided by AKC Parent Breed Clubs. Their contributions often cover up to 50 percent of a research request.

"Donor Advised Funds" are also accepted by the Foundation. These are donations restricted to research directed toward a specific breed or area. They typically come from the AKC Parent Breed Clubs. These donations are often invested in the manner of an endowment, growing in value and accumulating interest for application to research on specific health problems of a breed. To date, the Foundation's Donor Advised Fund program has been used by more than 50 breed clubs.

## Heritage Society

The Foundation's planned giving program is called the Heritage Society. Planned gifts of charitable remainder annuity trusts, real estate, art work, stock or other items of value can all qualify an individual for Heritage Society membership.

No matter what size the contribution, all donations support the accumulation of the knowledge necessary to promote health and well-being for our beloved canine companions who continually supply us with a bounty of joy and contentment.

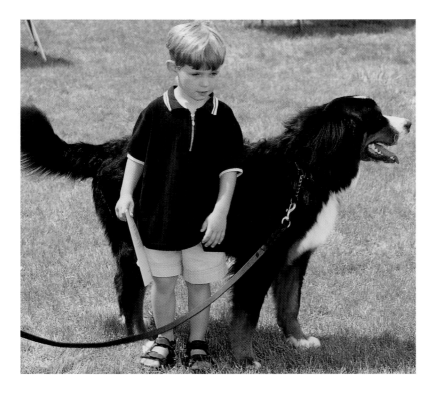

*Two of the four breeds of Swiss Mountain Dogs (Bernese and Greater Swiss) are shown in AKC competitions. All four were developed as drovers, draft and watch dogs on farms in the midlands of Switzerland. Faithful and hardy companions, they are well-suited for cold weather environs.*

# *Index*

# Index